THE DRY EYE
REMEDY

THE DRY EYE REMEDY

The Complete Guide to Restoring the Health and Beauty of Your Eyes

ROBERT LATKANY, M.D.
FOUNDER AND DIRECTOR OF
THE DRY EYE CLINIC
AT THE NEW YORK EYE & EAR INFIRMARY

HatherleighPress

New York • London

Hatherleigh Press
5-22 46th Avenue, Suite 200
Long Island City, NY 11101
www.hatherleighpress.com

DISCLAIMER
The ideas and suggestions contained in this book are not intended as a substitute for consulting with a physician. All matters regarding your health require medical supervision. Names of medications are typically followed by ™ or ® symbols, but these symbols are not stated in this book. The names of people who contributed anecdotal material have been changed.

Library of Congress Cataloging-in-Publication Data is available.

ISBN-13: 978-1-57826-242-7
ISBN-10: 1-57826-242-9

The Dry Eye Remedy is available for bulk purchase, special promotions, and premiums. For information on reselling and special purchase opportunities, call 1-800-528-2550 and ask for the Special Sales Manager.

Cover design by Level C
Interior design by Deborah Miller, Jasmine Cardoza, and Allison Furrer

10 9 8 7 6 5 4 3
Printed in the United States

DEDICATION

To my wife, Barbara

With thanks for putting up with all that pillow talk
about dry eye

Every day is still like the first day we met.

By special arrangement with the publisher, the author will donate a portion of the proceeds from the sales of this book to the Sjögren's Syndrome Foundation and to the Society for Women's Health Research to increase awareness of dry eye and to expand information on potential therapies.

ACKNOWLEDGMENTS

I n writing *The Dry Eye Remedy*, I have learned the extent to which authorship is a collaborative process, so I am pleased to be able to declare my gratitude to the many people who helped make this book possible.

First and foremost, I would like to thank my patients for indirectly encouraging me to establish myself as a dry eye specialist. The experience of treating suffering patients enabled me to perfect the detailed history, examination, and treatment regime for all types of dry eye sufferers. Dry eye is not a condition taught in medical school, and it receives little emphasis in residency training, so it is my patients who really taught me about this condition.

Thanks to Dr. Vickery Trinkaus-Randall for allowing me to be a part of her ophthalmic research team; I hope others will also benefit from such generosity. I am grateful to Dr. Celso Tello and Dr. Joseph Walsh for seeing potential in me and allowing me to train at the New York Eye & Ear Infirmary. To those who believed early on in my passion for treating dry eye, I thank Dr. Monica Lorenzo, Dr. Mark Kupersmith, Dr. Julius Schulman, Dr. Paul Finger, Dr. John Seedor, Dr. Jodi Abramson, Dr. Steven Ali, Dr. Arkady Selenow, Dr. Ann Abadir, and Dr. Robert Ritch for all their dry eye patient referrals. And I thank Dr. Mark Speaker for taking me under his wing and trusting me to pursue the "never been done before" career of a dry eye specialist.

I am grateful to Susanna Margolis for her editorial help—particularly impressive for someone who started off with no knowledge of the subject matter. To my agent Sarah Jane Freymann, it was not just a coincidence that we met: I thank you for seeing the potential in this book.

I am grateful also to the folks at Hatherleigh Press—editorial director Andrea Au and publisher Kevin Moran—for their support and for playing an active role in the book's development.

I would like to thank my mother Regina and my father Robert for being there for me every day. It is unfortunate that not everyone can be so lucky as to have parents like mine. I still remember every night that they put me to bed and said "pleasant dreams." I want also to thank my brother, Dr. Paul Latkany, without whose guidance and support I probably would never have been a physician. And I want my brother Joe and sisters Lianne and Lauren to know what a joy it was to be the youngest in our family. To my father-in-law Jim and mother-in-law Carolyn, I offer fondest appreciation of your encouragement and guidance.

Special thanks to my Uncle Adam, who not only introduced me to the game of golf but, more importantly, taught me the importance of generosity. I am sorry I never got a chance to say thank you, but I think about him every day since the day he passed.

To my beautiful children, Brian and Amanda—and those that may come—you bring a smile to my face whenever I see you. So please stay close by. I hope you will be as passionate about your career as I am about mine.

C O N T E N T S

INTRODUCTION

What's the Big Deal About Dry Eyes?

An estimated 30 percent of adult Americans are afflicted with dry eye, a disorder that adversely affects the tear film, which is the essential coating that protects the surface of the eye, washes away debris and irritants, and creates a crystal-clear window through which we see.

Those tens of millions of dry eye sufferers are the tip of the iceberg. For it is considered likely if not inevitable that everyone will experience the discomfort, irritation, displeasing appearance, and potential visual blurring of dry eye disorder at some point in their lives—if they haven't already.

In other words, we're all susceptible, and the categories of people deemed particularly susceptible are as wide-ranging as the population. Contact lens wearers, people with allergies, peri-menopausal women, people who have undergone laser eye surgery or cosmetic eye surgery: all of these—and others—may be said to be especially prone to dry eye disorder.

But...

Do you work in front of a computer all day? Spend your evenings glued to the television set? Have difficulty reading even a page-turner of a novel or your local newspaper? Find that you need a new prescription for your eyeglasses every two years? Notice that the whites of your eyes are kind of red?

Chances are good you have or will develop dry eye.

Do your eyes sometimes feel "gritty"? Are they crusty in the morning till you have your shower? Are there bags under your eyes that make you look a lot older than you are?

These, too, are symptoms of dry eye.

There's one certainty about these symptoms: untreated, they will only get worse. For dry eye is a progressive disorder. In fact, one reason we are hearing so much more about it today is that the first wave of Baby Boomers is just now coming into its 60s and just now beginning to feel the effects of dry eye, and the legendary refusal of the Boomer generation to accept the effects of growing older is often expressed vocally and loudly. Since the elderly are the fastest-growing population sector in the country, that decibel level is unlikely to go down any time soon.

The lesson, however, is clear: Don't wait. Don't put off treatment of dry eye till you're ready to scream along with the Baby Boomers. Whatever your age, you would be wise to start now to deal with the symptoms of dry eye. Begin today to do the things that can make you feel and look better so you break the back of this disorder before it robs you of vision or ages the appearance of your eyes well before time—and while it's still relatively easy for treatment to make a difference.

For while there is as yet no cure for dry eye, there are many, many options for dealing with the disorder so as to keep the eyes as healthy and youthful—looking as possible.

That's what this book is about.

Symptoms and Effects

Dry eye is almost a stealth disorder. Your eyes are tired, or they feel irritated, or they're looking red-and you tend not to give it a second thought. You suppose it's normal, and you get yourself some drops from the drugstore and forget all about it.

You shouldn't. Eye discomfort is not normal, and what you assess as minor irritation could be a signal of a deeper disorder or could grow into a major problem. Sensations of stinging, burning, grittiness, and itching in the eyes; sensitivity to light; the feeling that there is something in the eye; soreness, redness, the inability to wear contact lenses for very long; an aged and wrinkled appearance and the area around the eyes: these may all be symptoms of dry eye disorder. All should be reported to your doctor. All should be dealt with medically—and all are most certainly covered by health insurance plans.

But dry eye is more than discomfort. The clinical term for what these symptoms represent is "thief of sight," as the instability the disorder causes to the eye's tear film impairs quality of vision bit by bit. At the same time, the disorder's intermittent but chronic irritation saps the person's energy and robs the body of its natural vigor. All of this can erode the individual's ability to read, drive at night, or even use the phone or an ATM machine.

It can also affect more than your eyes. One patient of mine, a high-level corporate executive I'll call Philip, told me his dry eye was such a persistent annoyance—so utterly preoccupying when he was trying to work—that he actually forgot the names of co-workers. Pain in the eye, after all, is pain you cannot get away from; it can be distracting, and it can affect your state of mind, your mood, and your productivity, as Philip's case makes clear.

Think about people who work all day in front of a computer screen—and there are more and more such people with every passing year. They're concentrating hard, focusing on the screen. And although the work may not be particularly stressful, by 3:00 in the afternoon, they feel exhausted, and the pace of their work ebbs, slows, then crashes to a halt. The problem? We tend to blink less when we concentrate. Less blinking means the tear film isn't coating and protecting the eye. Result: you feel tired, you soon can't concentrate, you lose focus—your productivity takes a nosedive. Can dry eye be blamed for lowered productivity in today's offices? For some of it, certainly.

Dry eye can also affect the way you look. You tend to rub your tired or irritated eyes. The rubbing exacerbates the irritation. You squint to get rid of the irritation. You look at yourself in the mirror and see lines, wrinkles, bags, redness that were never there before.

Or maybe you're an allergy sufferer—and the number of allergy sufferers, so great as to be impossible to estimate, continues to increase. Allergies tend to locate in the eyes, where they cause inflammation. Unhappily, most anti-allergy medicines only worsen the dry eye dysfunction. Result? Allergy sufferers rub their eyes almost automatically; over the long term, this stretches and wrinkles the skin, causing a telltale old-eyes look.

No one wants to look that way. No one wants to feel the tiredness, irritation, and discomfort that dry eye produces. And certainly no one wants to neglect the health of their eyes such that they may damage their appearance, feel chronic discomfort, or imperil their vision.

You don't have to.

Dry Eye and Me

My experience with dry eye is both personal and professional. I was diagnosed with the disorder when I was in my early 20s, so I can empathize, virtually symptom for symptom, with other dry eye sufferers. But it's what I've seen as a practicing ophthalmologist that has prompted me to specialize exclusively in dry eye—and to write this book.

I've seen this pervasive disorder affect people's lives in profound ways, and I've seen it all too often go unnoticed, undiagnosed or under-diagnosed, unmanaged and under-treated.

A patient I'll call Bill came to my office after getting his sixth new eyeglass prescription in seven years. After spending $500 per new pair of glasses, Bill's wallet was feeling as deprived as Bill was feeling befuddled. Bill told me that his vision sometimes turned blurry—"I can be reading the paper, and suddenly it'll go all blurry on me," he said, but it would then just as suddenly return to "normal."

Bill assumed that his fluctuating vision was a matter of visual acuity; in fact, it sounded to me like a typical symptom of dry eye. It wasn't an imperfect prescription that was blurring his vision; it was something altering the state of the tear film that coats the surface of the eye. I performed my proprietary diagnostic test and found that to be the case. Bill's blurry vision was due to just such a dysfunction on the surface of his eye, not to the state of his eyesight. At least five of his new eyeglasses had probably been unnecessary; as long as his dry eye went untreated, his vision would never be truly "corrected." But a simple course of treatments, such as you'll read in the pages that follow, solved Bill's vision problem and potentially stalled the decline in the health of his eyes.

Emily had undergone LASIK surgery five years ago, but now the sharpness of her vision was starting to slip just a bit, and she was contemplating "touch-up" surgery. Still, Emily knew that any kind of surgical procedure presented the possibility of side effects, so she asked for a second opinion and was referred to my office.

This was a sensible move on Emily's part—and to some extent, a surprising one; so many patients who have undergone the expense and trouble of surgery simply want their surgeons to "fix it." This is perhaps a natural reaction: patients who choose LASIK often think they are buying perfection, although perfection is rarely possible. Emily's willingness to consider alternative approaches was both refreshing and smart. Together, we decided to try an alternative course of treatment first, and I designed a series of simple therapies to improve Emily's vision by improving her ocular surface. The safer alternatives worked, and Emily saved herself both the expense and the potential risks of further surgery.

Dan told me his boss had ordered him to "see an eye doctor." Dan's eyes were intermittently bloodshot; the boss's view was that Dan was "out partying too much" and would soon be unable to work productively. For the wrong reason, the boss was right: Dan's eyes were angry-looking and red, not from late nights on the town, but from the chronic irritation dry eye can produce. Untreated, Dan's eye condition would indeed soon lower his productivity as his feelings of fatigue and discomfort increased. But with simple treatment, we were able to decrease the irritation in Dan's eyes, which in turn cleared up the redness, which made Dan feel invigorated and enabled him to work in a highly productive manner. It also convinced his boss that he was a sober and serious young man and a conscientious employee.

Bill, Emily, and Dan are just some of the reasons why I now see only patients with symptoms related to dry eye—because I can make a difference in the way they feel and look and in the long-term health of their eyes. In fact, although I have performed perhaps a thousand laser eye and cataract surgeries, I no longer do so; I treat dry eye exclusively.

I also lecture on the subject, publish frequently, present findings on dry eye both nationally and internationally, serve on panels on the subject at medical conferences, and sit on advisory committees for related conditions.

Over the years, I have treated dry eye disorders of varying intensity and deriving from varied first causes. I have devised my own classifications for the many, varied effects of dry eye, have created my own diagnostic test for the disorder—which is gaining ground as a possible standard for ophthalmologists around the country—and have even designed a set of eye care products specifically for dry eye sufferers.

I've used traditional treatments and pioneered new ones to alleviate the discomfort, manage the disease, and treat the disorder. I know how to help patients deal with dry eye so that they feel and look better—and so that they improve the health of their eyes.

That's my message, and now I want to bring it to a wider audience. Hence this book.

The Goal: Not a Dry Eye in the House

My aim has been to offer a complete handbook to the disorders of the eye surface and how to deal with them. The book is aimed not just at those who know they are afflicted with dry eye but also at those who are concerned about the health of their eyes and want to know what they can do to improve it. For the health of your eyes is the real issue.

That's why Part One begins with a discussion of healthy eyes and how they work, so that when you then learn what can go wrong, you will understand how dry eye affects the health of your eyes and what it may mean for your overall health.

You'll also learn here how you can work with your doctor to find the precise origin of your dry eye disorder and to come up with the best course of action for treating your symptoms. So many other factors affect your eyes—allergies, contact lenses, the medicines you may be taking for another health condition, to name just a few—that it is essential to draw a complete picture of your eye health before you proceed to treatment. Part One of the book ends with a discussion of how dry eye has traditionally been treated—and the limits of those traditional treatments.

Part Two presents my own program for restoring the health

of your dry eyes. Here you'll find adjustments you can make in your environment—home, workplace, even in your car—and tips for nutrition and lifestyle that can bring substantial relief from the discomforts of dry eye while helping to keep your eyes as healthy as possible. In addition, you'll learn here my Home Eye Spa procedure—a simple but highly effective cleansing and soothing procedure you can do at home. It's a way of both gaining immediate relief and taking direct responsibility for the long-term health of your eyes.

In Part Three, you'll learn about the growing list of medicines for dry eye—those that can help and those that might harm—and about other kinds of interventions to treat the disorder, including the potential for hormone therapy, punctal plugs, and surgery.

Finally, I'll put it all together for you in Part Four by profiling some typical courses of therapy that encompass the state of the art for treating dry eye disorders today. These are programs that have worked well for my patients and that, in one form or another, may work well for you.

At the back of the book, you'll also find a list of resources you can turn to for more information or for direct help with your dry eye disorder or related conditions.

Some of you may find that there is too much detail in the early chapters that explain the workings of the healthy eye and the origins of dry eye disorder, or that the discussion is too technical. Others, of course, will assess the book as not technical or detailed enough. There are tens of millions of dry eye sufferers out there, and I have tried to strike a middle path to reach as many of you as possible. Certainly, whatever your tolerance for technical detail, you all want the same thing: a better way to relieve your dry eye discomfort and improve the health of your eyes.

But there is yet another reason for this book. Incurable, progressive, potentially damaging to vision, uncomfortable, disfiguring, and psychologically distressing for its impact on the individual's abilities and appearance, dry eye constitutes a debilitating and harmful condition, and when 30 percent of the adult population suffers a debilitating and harmful condition, in my view, that is nothing short of a public health problem.

I hope this book will raise awareness of the problem among patients, doctors, and the general population, which, as the number of elderly grows, will increasingly be at risk for dry eye. Remember: the one thing we know for sure about this disorder is that if you do nothing, it will get worse. Even if you are in your twenties or thirties with mild symptoms, it is easier and certainly more effective to establish a treatment therapy or maintenance regime now than twenty years from now, when the condition may be far more severe. So now is the time to act, and in the pages that follow, I hope you will find the understanding and information you need to create an action plan that is right for you.

Robert Latkany, M.D.
New York, 2007

PART ONE

UNDERSTANDING DRY EYE DISORDERS

Since it's hard to appreciate what can go wrong with your eyes until you understand how your eyes work when everything is going right, Part One begins by showing you what constitutes healthy eyes. You'll learn the basic components of the eye and how all the parts work together in a brilliant system that brings the entire world into your consciousness. The danger is that if something goes wrong with any one of the moving parts, the entire system can be adversely affected, and you'll learn in Chapter 2 just exactly what can go wrong and how your eye health and your vision may be affected.

You'll also learn how eye doctors diagnose dry eye—the tests they use and what they are looking for—so that you can communicate knowledgeably with your eye health care provider. Your doctor may recommend a range of over-the-counter treatments as a first step toward dealing with your dry eye, or you may have browsed the drugstore shelves for help even before consulting a doctor. These popular treatments have a range of uses and effects, and Part One ends by articulating the purpose of each, its benefits, and its potential limits.

1

How Healthy Eyes Work

Have you ever tried not blinking? Try it now: don't blink for 20 seconds. Look at your watch, and as the seconds tick by, concentrate hard on keeping your eyes open. Ready? Go.

It's virtually impossible, isn't it? After just a few seconds of holding your eyes open, they feel gritty and uncomfortable. Keep it up, and they begin to sting with irritation. In fact, even if you think you haven't blinked in 20 seconds, chances are you have.

In a way, the reason for this is simple: keeping your eyes open dries them out, and the naturally healthy state of the eyes is wet. Blinking is the eye's mechanism for staying wet; the rapid closing and opening of the eyelid coat the eye with a film of tears. When you will yourself not to blink, the tear film doesn't get produced, and the ocular surface, instantly uncomfortable, sends a message of dryness to the brain. Reflexively, the brain responds by "commanding" the eye to blink, triggering the tear film to start flowing again and re-moisten the eye.

In another way, however, this response to the need for moisture isn't simple at all. In fact, it's very complicated, based in an intricate and highly integrated system for producing and maintaining tear film. When all the myriad parts of the system work together perfectly, the tear film flows as it should, continually refreshing the eye surface and keeping it healthy. That's important, because a healthy ocular surface is what keeps your vision sharp, your eyes infection-free, and the cells on the surface of your eye alive and well. Put it this way: a wet ocular surface is a healthy ocular surface, and a healthy ocular surface is one of the keys to overall eye health and good vision.

The problem occurs if and when any part of this intricate, integrated system breaks or becomes disrupted or gets destabilized in some way, for even the tiniest deviation will affect the whole system, drying the ocular surface. And precisely because the system is so complex, with so many moving parts, any number of factors can cause such a break or disruption or destabilization. The resulting disorder—and there's a whole range of disorders associated with dry eye—will be bad for your vision and bad for the health of your eyes.

How can you keep the tear film in your eyes flowing regularly so that the ocular surface is continually bathed in restoring moisture—and so that you avoid the damaging disorders of dry eye? That's what this book is all about. It's the toolkit for a healthy ocular surface—itself the prerequisite for healthy eyes and clear vision. It will tell you how to prevent dry eye where possible and how to treat it where necessary.

You'll have a lot of help in doing so. The whole structure of the eye, as we'll see shortly, and all sorts of mechanisms inside it are geared toward keeping the ocular surface moist. Understanding why and how that's so is essential to understanding how you can prevent dry eye and/or deal with it should it occur. Awareness, after all, is the first step toward good health, so let's take a look at how the ocular surface works and how all the moving parts of the system operate together.

What Is Tear Film?

Peel an onion…watch a sappy movie…experience profound grief or thrilling elation…and there probably won't be a dry eye in the house. The tears come pouring out—first squeezed out as drops, then in rivulets, all absolutely automatically.

The tear film on the ocular surface, however, is not an occasional event caused by a very specific stimulation; it's just there, all the time. And it's not a gushing waterfall like tears of grief or onion tears; it is an actual film that coats the ocular surface and is constantly being replenished.

The tear film consists of three distinct layers. Once upon a time, scientists believed those layers were placed one atop the other, like a deli sandwich. Now, we think the three are intermixed—more like a pâté than a sandwich—although each still has its own character and its own purpose:

- The oily layer of tear film acts as a protective shield helping prevent evaporation—particularly evaporation of another layer of tear film, the watery or aqueous layer.
- The aqueous layer contains a variety of important proteins. These include antibacterial proteins that fight infection,

growth factor proteins that help heal wounds and promote the equilibrium of the system, even proteins called immunoglobulins that combat foreign bodies—all creating what is, in effect, a critical defense mechanism. The aqueous layer makes up the majority of the tear film.

- The mucous layer of the tear film creates the nice, even spread of the film across the ocular surface, distributing the tears evenly so they don't funnel away from the surface too quickly.

Each layer is critical to the others; together, they form and maintain the tear film that protects the surface of the eye, nourishes the eye, and of course refracts light so you can see nice, sharp images.

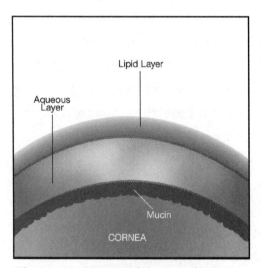

Figure 1: *Layers of the tear film*

The Lacrimal Gland Functional Unit

What continually creates the tear film and makes it all work is a system we call the lacrimal gland functional unit. It consists of a set of glands scattered around the surface of the eye—three different sets of glands, in fact—a special category of cells, and a network of nerves and muscles that gets the unit moving. Let's take them one at a time.

Glands are simply structures that produce secretions, and lacrimal glands produce the secretions that create the eye's tear film. ("Lacrima" is Latin for tear.) A gland called the main gland is responsible for reflex tears, the tears that are automatic reactions to an irritant or stimulation. The tears you shed when you peel that onion, or watch the sappy movie, or experience great grief or joy, are reflex tears, pumped out as watery tear film by the main gland.

The basic, everyday portion of the tear film—the routine tears that are on the ocular surface whether there's an onion handy or not—come from accessory lacrimal glands, and these tears too are pumped out as an aqueous substance.

Right along your eyelid margin on both the upper and lower eyelid—although occurring in greater proportion in the upper eyelid—are the so-called meibomian glands, some 50 of them, that pump out the oily layer of the tear film.

In addition to the glands, a class of cells called goblet cells is essential to the lacrimal gland functional unit. The special talent of goblet cells, wherever they occur in the body, is to pump out mucus. In the eye, these cells are scattered around what is called the conjunctiva, the thin, transparent tissue that covers the white of the eye. It's there that the goblet cells secrete the mucous layer of the tear film.

The last component of the lacrimal gland functional unit is the neuromuscular component—the nerves and muscles that get the unit functioning. When the nerve endings in the cornea and conjunctiva of the ocular surface sense dryness, they send a reflex to the brain. The brain in turn sends a reflex back to the muscles of the eye, triggering a blink—and the accessory glands, meibomian glands, and goblet cells start pumping out the layers of the tear film again.

THE BLINK OF AN EYE

This complex functional unit, which evolved specifically to protect the surface of the eye, is behind every blink of your eye, although, of course, it all works pretty much beyond your awareness. Indeed, unless you make a conscious effort to think about it, you're totally unaware that you've blinked.

For one thing, it all takes place in a unit of time too small to measure. The sensation of dryness happens very fast. In fact, the cornea has the single highest concentration of nerve endings of any structure in the body. So it takes very little time for it to feel discomfort and set in motion the sequence of reflexes that makes us blink.

Once the blinking gets underway, it initiates what is basically a process of drainage and refill. The process operates through a system of minuscule drainage tubes controlled by valves, and it works on the principle of positive and negative pressure—just the way some heat transfer or ventilation systems work. The drainage tubes, the opening of which is called a punctum, are located right in the lower and upper eyelids near the nose. The location is significant, because our tear film drains through the punctum into the nose. (Yes, that's why your nose runs when you cry.) It also connects to your throat, which is why you can actually taste some eye drops after you've applied them to your eyes. Here's how it all works when a healthy eye blinks:

In the eye-closing portion of the blink, the closing action pushes the tears collected in the punctal tubes, and the positive pressure contracts the muscles and forces open the valves. Result? The tears drain out the tubes into your nose. When the eye then opens to complete the blink, the opening action—negative pressure—sucks the tears from the ocular surface back into the tubes, so that you're again ready for a blink.

It's true that a small portion of tears evaporate from the ocular surface, but the majority by far drain through the punctal ducts, which empty and fill as the pressure changes open and close their valves.

But of course, it all happens in the blink of an eye.

A Brilliant Design, Except When Things Go Wrong…

In one sense, the ocular surface is brilliantly designed. With its myriad moisture-producing glands and cells—including a vital supply of stem cells that continually regenerate cells that die—its system of tubes and valves, the network of nerves and muscles that make it all go, it's a superbly effective structure for maintaining the eye's moisture. This protects the ocular surface and keeps vision sharp.

But in another sense, the very genius of the design is also its weakness. Because every component of the system is essential to the whole, the slightest deviation or alteration or destabilization can disrupt the lacrimal functional unit, diminish the efficiency of the blink, and compromise the overall health of the eye and the overall quality of your vision.

How can it affect vision? Think about it: the ocular surface is

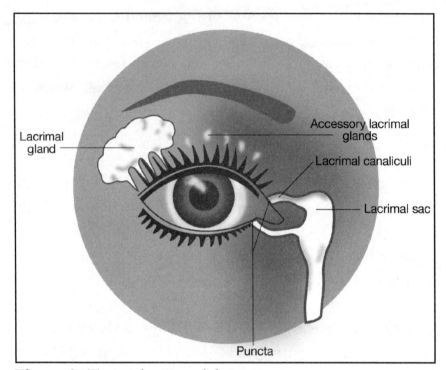

Figure 2: *Tear production and drainage system*

the front of the eye—like the outside pane of glass in a window. So even if the rest of your eye is perfectly healthy, the slightest "smudge" on that outside pane will affect how well you see.

And a dry eye can put you at risk for anything from a slight infection to loss of vision. And the truth is that despite all the protection of the ocular surface—including the eyelashes, which keep foreign bodies out of the eye and moisture in—it really doesn't take much to create the conditions in which infection can occur.

To understand this, it may help to remember what it's like when you have chapped lips. Indeed, it's much the same process, because the surface of the lips is a mucous membrane much like the tear film on the ocular surface. When dry winter weather, or over-exposure to the sun, or even vitamin deficiencies dry out this mucous membrane, it quite literally splits; the membrane simply breaks down. Bacteria can easily enter these splits in the membrane, which is why chapped lips can range from an uncomfortably rough surface to cracked, badly infected lips that bleed easily and are extremely painful.

The same thing can happen with the eye if the ocular surface breaks down: bacteria can intrude into the surface and cause an infection. The worse the hole in the ocular surface, the more profound the infection.

The problem is that with so many moving parts—glands, cells, tubes, valves, nerves, muscles, etc.—any number of things can go wrong, and anything that goes wrong can start to break down the ocular surface. In other words, the very complexity that is the wonder of the ocular surface is also its potential bane, because it means there are many ways to disrupt the system and destabilize the eye's surface.

To translate that into medical terms, those of us who treat dry eye say that it is a multifactorial disorder—one that is caused by any of several factors. And that is also why there is no one-size-fits-all treatment that can be applied to the disorder. On the contrary: we need to find out the precise point of origin of the problem in order to address an individual's particular form of dry eye. That means determining exactly which part of the system has been destabilized or needs repair.

A patient I'll call Angela offers a perfect example of this.

Angela suffers from a not uncommon situation: she sleeps with her eyes ever so slightly open. This condition, said to affect some five to 10 percent of the population—my guess is that it affects many more than that—is known as lagophthalmos. (The name comes from the Greek words for "rabbit eyes," because rabbits are said to sleep with their eyes open.) Needless to say, lagophthalmos adversely affects the quality of the person's night sleep, and sleep deprivation over long periods of time becomes physically and emotionally damaging.

It's also a sure-fire way to develop dry eye disorder. The reason? For the eyes, as for the rest of the body, sleep represents a time of repair and restoration. Where the eyes are concerned, that requires total closure: the upper eyelid must meet the lower eyelid and in effect seal the eye so that it bathes in its own protective healthy tear film, without the drying and evaporative effects of "outside" air. If you've ever pulled an all-nighter, that's why your eyes felt so tired and gritty the next day—because they never had the chance to restore themselves in that moist, airtight environment. Lagophthalmos sufferers pull repeated one-nighters, in a manner of speaking, and the extended exposure of the eyes can create scratch marks and dry spots on the eye surface that over time can lead to blood vessel growth and scarring—and eventually, to possible loss of function and of vision. I frequently astonish patients by informing them for the first time of something they find hard to believe: that they sleep with their eyes open. Most go home, check with their spouse, and report back that I'm wrong; they maintain that view until we begin the therapy for lagophthalmos. Then they're convinced that I was right.

But knowing that Angela suffered from the condition was only the beginning. It was then essential to find out why her eyes do not fully close during sleep. Is it a result of some sort of paralysis? Is it hereditary? Are her eye muscles losing tensile strength as Angela ages? Had she had cosmetic surgery? The latter, as it turned out, was indeed the source of Angela's lagophthalmos, and knowing that enabled me to devise a course of treatment that would be effective because it addressed the exact reason for the

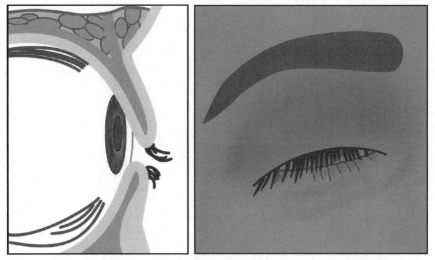

Figure 3: *Examples of lagophthalmos, the inability to fully close the eyelids*

disruption to her ocular surface. The typical treatment for dry eye—artificial tears and liquid drops—addresses inflammation as the cause of the dryness; that would clearly not have worked for Angela. The treatment I prescribed for her, by contrast, addressed her core problem, nighttime exposure, and used a combination of ophthalmic ointments and a nighttime eye mask made specifically for lagophthalmos sufferers. The prescription quickly brought her the relief she sought.

But Angela's story points up the importance of identifying the exact nature of dry eye and its precise cause. That's why it's essential for you to understand how a healthy ocular surface works, and why and how things can go wrong with it. Only in that way can you truly help your doctor address the root of the problem and create a course of treatment that will work to end your discomfort and protect your vision.

2

WHAT CAUSES DRY EYE DISORDERS?

It's worth repeating: precisely because the structure and mechanisms of the ocular surface are so complex, just about anything can upset the delicate balance that keeps your eyes moist and healthy. If the lacrimal glands, meibomian glands, or goblet cells are in some way adversely affected, that can break down the tear film and lead to dry eye. Similarly, anything that alters your blink rate or your ability to close your eyes fully—in other words, any injury or harm to the nerves or muscles—can also lead to an unhealthy or unstable tear film and dry eye symptoms.

In short, any number of causes or triggers can destabilize the tear film. But whatever the trigger or underlying cause, when things do go wrong, one of two things happens:

1. An increased rate of evaporation of the tear film, or
2. A decreased rate of production of the tear film.

In other words, your eyes may be losing moisture faster than it can be replaced, or they may not be making enough moisture.

Moreover, this isn't necessarily an either/or proposition. Your eyes might be doing both—losing moisture too fast and not creating enough new moisture—at the same time.

By far the most common causes of these destabilizations of the tear film are simple enough—your contact lenses are bothering you, or you have allergies, or you're a post-menopausal woman, or you're simply growing older. But there are also a number of diseases and conditions of which dry eye is a byproduct-and which dry eye can signal—so it's important for dry eye sufferers to be aware of the possible causes of the disorder. Most of the evidence, in fact, points to inflammation as the likely "original" antecedent of the triggers causing dry eye disorder. (You can read much more about this in Chapter 6.)

So let's take a look first at some of the more common causes of evaporative loss.

Evaporation Through Meibomian Gland Dysfunction

Remember the meibomian glands? They're the 50 or so minute glands in your eyelids that pump out the oily layer of the tear film, known as the meibum. Since oil floats on water, the meibum exists precisely to protect against evaporation of the tear film's watery layer. Naturally, any malfunction in the meibomian glands will adversely affect the oily layer of the tear film, and even the slightest deterioration in the amount or quality of the oily layer will expose the aqueous layer of the tear film to evaporation. And one of the most common causes of meibomian gland dysfunction isn't something most people connect with the eyes at all. Instead, it's a condition generally thought of as a skin disease.

June was 29 years old and had complained of redness and irritation in her eyes for a long time. A range of doctors had treated her with a range of therapies, but nothing worked. She had been told she had dry eye, but nobody had been able to tell her why—or what might be causing it.

When I walked into the examining room where June was waiting, I was immediately struck, from 10 feet away, by the contrast between her clear, pale complexion and the redness of her eyes. Let me say here and now that I always look closely at patients' faces and eyes when I first meet them, as I search their facial anatomy, watch them blink, and note how they look back at me for clues about their vision and eye health. The first thought that came into my mind on seeing June was that there had to be a reason for the redness, which was so much at odds with her complexion. As I drew closer to her, I noticed some unevenness of the skin around her nose, above her eyebrow, and along her chin. And by the time I was close enough to shake hands with her, it was clear that June's face was covered with heavy pancake make-up. It was well done; the make-up had produced a rather silky matte "finish" that made her complexion look soft, even silky, from a distance. But the make-up had clearly been applied to cover something up.

"You're wearing make-up," I said to June. "I wonder what your face looks like without it."

"It's red and blotchy," June replied without skipping a beat, "with lots of blood vessels and small pimples all over. I'm a wreck."

What June was describing were the classic signs of rosacea, an increasingly common chronic disease affecting some 14 million Americans, many of whom don't know they have the disorder. Characterized by the deep-red flushing that typically affects the whole center of the face, rosacea is a major cause of dry eye as well. The angry blood vessels that cause the redness in the facial skin are usually repeated in the white of the eye—exactly what was happening with June. The presence of those blood vessels typically means that something has irritated and inflamed the vessels and that inflammatory cells are leaking out. In the eyes, that signals a dysfunction of the meibomian glands. Indeed, in June's case, when I gently pressed her eyelids, it was like popping a row of pimples, as the pressure loosened a viscous yellow pus containing the inflammatory cells from the tiny glands in her lids.

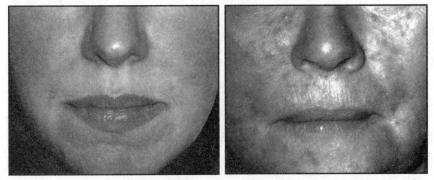

Figure 4: *Examples of the facial redness, left, and bumps and pimples, right, typical of rosacea*

Needless to say, understanding that June's dry eye was due to a dysfunction of the meibomian glands—and knowing further that the dysfunction was a result of a dermatological condition—meant that I could work with her skin doctor to create an effective course of treatment. Here's confirmation again that not all dry eye conditions are the same, that different dry eye disorders respond differently to different treatments, and that identifying the first cause that triggers dry eye is absolutely essential if the treatment is to be effective.

There are other causes of meibomian gland dysfunction; for example, the evidence is growing that the hormone components in the eyelid may in some way cause dry eye, as you'll read in greater detail in Chapter 9. And a condition known as blepharitis is also suspect, as you'll learn more about in Chapter 10. And not every patient with meibomian gland dysfunction suffers from rosacea. But virtually everyone who has rosacea almost surely has dry eye on occasion, whether they know it or not. It's ironic as well as unfortunate that in this case, those rosy red cheeks are not a sign of good health but rather of a very sensitive skin disorder that typically also brings the suffering of dry eye.

Evaporation through Failure of the Blink Mechanism

Both the number of times you blink and the completeness or incompleteness of the blink are essential factors in preventing evaporation of the tear film or failing to prevent it. Anything that disrupts the normal blink rate or keeps the eyelid from closing entirely is going to lead to rapid evaporation of the tear film—and the ensuing symptoms of dry eye.

What's a normal blink rate? For the most part, the answer is as individual as a fingerprint; some people blink fast, and some blink slowly. A study on the subject of blink rates in healthy eyes shows a range of rates—from a very low rate on average of 4.5 blinks per minute when an individual reads, to a very high rate of 26 during an animated conversation, settling down to a mean at-rest rate of about 17 blinks on average per minute. If your normal at-rest blink rate is every 5 seconds, therefore, and something happens to make you blink every 12 seconds instead, then you are not blinking often enough to spread your tear film adequately over your eye, and the tear film is going to evaporate much more rapidly. Result? It won't be long before you're feeling the symptoms of dry eye.

But blink rate isn't the only important factor; equally critical is whether your blink is complete or partial. If you only manage

What's Your Blink Rate?

Want to know how often you blink? Recruit a friend to do the counting, and ask him or her to do it in two different situations—and when you have no idea it is going on. First, the friend should count the number of times you blink when you're doing something that requires concentration—like reading. Then, the friend should take a second count when you're not concentrating. Remember: both counts must be taken at times that you are unaware you are being metered. How do your blink rates compare to the average blink rates of the healthy eyes noted above? If your blink rates are less frequent, that might indicate that the ocular surface is not being moistened frequently enough.

a partial blink, you're leaving part of your eye open and therefore exposed to evaporative forces. I've seen patients whose eyelids only close three-quarters of the way down. As you'd expect, the upper three-quarters of their eyes are healthy; the bottom quarters are dry. To check for this at home, pull down your lower eyelid or pull up your upper eyelid and check the white part of your eye. If the white part that is exposed looks relatively pink or red, it may be an indication of a partial or incomplete blink.

SLOW BLINK RATES

What can affect the rate of blinking? A number of diseases slow the blink rate markedly.

Diabetes, for example, reduces the individual's neural sensation capability, and that affects the nerve endings in the eyes as well. The ocular surface of a diabetic's eye is typically covered with tiny scratch marks that appear sharply incised and with a very unstable tear film—a telltale appearance of this disease to any eye doctor—yet due to the loss of sensitivity of the nerve endings, the diabetic could not sense the damage when it was being inflicted and cannot sense its aftereffects now. By the same token, the nerve endings in the eyes of many diabetics are slow to sense dryness; they don't send that message telling the brain to instruct the muscles to blink and make more tearsso dryness results.

Herpes zoster (also known as shingles) is another common disease that can alter the blink mechanism. Herpes is a nerve infection, and one of the classic areas for it to establish residence is the eye. There, the herpes zoster creates an inflammation of the nerves, reducing sensation and thus, as with diabetes, shutting off the blink reflex. As a consequence, herpes zoster patients typically become chronic dry eye sufferers.

LASIK (Laser–assisted in situ keratomileusis) surgery, the most popular form of laser eye surgery, requires severing more than 70 percent of the superficial corneal nerves. The surgeon creates a flap on the cornea of the eye, then cuts down into the cornea itself, severing nerve endings in both places. Next, the surgeon lifts the flap, lasers the remaining bed of the cornea to the proper prescription, then lowers the flap back down. The procedure is popular because the flap acts as a kind of bandage, and as a result, patients regain a level of comfort quite soon— usually by the next day. But severing the nerve endings greatly reduces patients' dryness reflexes. So they won't blink as much as they used to, or as much as they should. Of course, the nerves regenerate over the course of time, reverting back to the baseline level after a few years.

In **PRK** (photorefractive keratectomy) and **LASEK** (laser epithelial keratomileusis) procedures, by contrast, the surgeon just scrapes the superficial skin layer off the eye, then lasers in the prescription. The eventual vision correction effect is the same as in LASIK—in fact, there is evidence that by the sixth month after surgery, it is actually superior. But because the surgeon need not create a flap nor cut as deep, far fewer nerve endings are cut, and the eyes of patients undergoing PRK or LASEK procedures tend to be a lot less dry. Moreover, although it can take from four to six days immediately following the procedure for these patients' eyes to regain a level of complete comfort and visual acuity, the eyes' nerve endings regenerate after about a year—sooner than with LASIK—and there is evidence as well that, six months after the procedure, overall visual acuity gets better than with LASIK and stays better. So patients considering laser eye surgery would do well to discuss all options with their eye doctor and/or surgeon, for the slowed blink rate that can result from these procedures may cause unpleasant and unhealthful eye dryness.

PARTIAL BLINKING

As for partial blinking, it too may be caused by a number of factors. Certain diseases, for example, may permanently shorten the blink.

People with any kind of **thyroid condition** get what is routinely called the "thyroid stare"; the condition itself increases the size of the eye muscles surrounding the eyes such that the eyeballs bulge, and the eyelids cannot fully close.

Bell's Palsy weakens one side of the face so that the patient cannot close the eye on that side, a condition that may last for months or forever.

Parkinson's patients are partial blinkers because of the neuromuscular impact of their disease. Do you remember the last time you saw Muhammed Ali on television? The motor system disorder is so advanced on this great athlete, that he seems not to blink at all; he simply stares, open-eyed, unable to close his eyelids.

Some partial blinkers are just born with **large eyeballs**; their eyelids simply cannot manage to cover the whole surface of the eye. These lagophthalmos sufferers typically are light sleepers, wake up with a crusty feeling around their eyes, and often can't seem to "wake up" till a nice hot shower has got them going— i.e., has moistened their eyes sufficiently. They may have no idea that they sleep with their eyes open, and I've often stunned new patients by announcing to them that that's the reason they feel tired in the mornings.

There's one more significant way the blink mechanism gets compromised: by staring. Perhaps you're a professional truck driver tooling down an interstate in heavy traffic and keeping a sharp eye out for smaller cars and other trucks…or you're a commodities trader watching five computer screens at once and determined not to miss a single upswing or downtick of the market…or you're a secretary typing in front of a computer all day. It won't take long before you feel the dryness settling into your unblinking eyes. Fortunately, unless you suffer from one of the diseases or disorders mentioned above, you will blink in due course, and once you stop staring, you can return your eyes to their normal blink rate and to full closure of the eyelids. But any deliberate and determined staring is a burden on your blink rate and can hasten the evaporation of your tear film. Avoid it if you can.

Decreased Tear Production

In the category of decreased tear production as a cause of dry eye, we must consider two sub-categories of causes: the disorder known as Sjögren's Syndrome, and everything else.

Sjögren's Syndrome

Sjögren's syndrome is a chronic, systemic disease that targets the body's moisture-producing glands, especially in the eyes and mouth. Sjögren's affects one percent of the female population of the United States—nearly four million people—and is the second most common rheumatologic autoimmune disease. In fact, it is associated with such other autoimmune conditions as rheumatoid arthritis, lupus, scleroderma, and dermatomyositis; these patients also typically suffer from joint pain. In Sjögren's syndrome, white blood cells called lymphocytes, normally part of the body's defense system against germs and foreign invaders, infiltrate the lacrimal glands. There, they take over a space and interrupt the tear-secreting process.

Sjögren's syndrome is an extremely debilitating condition that must be diagnosed by a combination of blood tests, biopsy, and examination of the symptoms of dry eye, dry mouth, and/or vaginal dryness. Typically, those who suffer from it have very severe cases of dryness. They may have difficulty swallowing and speaking and often contract oral infections; they also usually suffer from an arthritic condition. Where the eyes are concerned, Sjögren's produces perhaps the worst level of dryness there is.

Unfortunately, there is no known cure for Sjögren's syndrome. For its dry eye effects, Sjögren's patients receive very aggressive treatment with very powerful anti-inflammatory medicine given orally, and they must continue it for their lifetime.

Other Causes of Decreased Tear Production

Just as you can be born with a condition that promotes evaporation of your tear film, it's possible to be born with some deficiency in the lacrimal gland itself, so that sufficient tears are not produced at the source. It is more likely, however, that other health conditions will cause a temporary or permanent infiltration of the glands that disrupts the production of tears. That, in turn, will lead to the symptoms of dry eye.

Again, it's worth remembering that the tear production mechanism works through a fine network of microscopic tubes, ducts, and glands. It doesn't take much for something to penetrate the network, where the slightest compression or scarring can lead to inflammation. A range of conditions can cause such infiltration.

Various **infections**, among them **hepatitis C, mononucleosis,** and **conjunctivitis** (or **pinkeye**), can disrupt the tear-secretion mechanism. I recently treated a 23-year-old woman with a severe case of dry eye. She seemed in all other respects to be entirely healthy, but the existence of pinpoint scratches on the ocular surface was alarming, especially since she was not a contact lens wearer. (Contact lens damage to the ocular surface is a major source of dry eye and pinpoint scratches are very common in contact lens wearers.) But in the case of this patient, the scratches signaled the possibility of infiltration of the lacrimal glands, so I ordered a range of tests. Both the patient and I were startled to discover that she was HIV-positive. She is doing well, but it was interesting—and in a way fortunate—that her dry eye presented the only evident symptoms of her infection.

Lymphomas can infiltrate the lacrimal glands as well, and the **radiation** used to treat so many cancers can, if targeted on or around the face, result in similar disruption of the tear secretion process.

In some cases, intensely **allergic reactions** to drugs—anything from the wrong eye drop to a course of antibiotics—can lead to scarring of the tear secretion mechanism in a way that literally alters the mechanism's function. In the most severe of these reactions, known as the **Stevens Johnson syndrome**, the body's reaction focuses on the mucous membranes of the eye and mouth. The inflammatory reaction is acute and devastating, and although it may pass, the scarring it has caused will have modified the tear production function so profoundly that it is permanently dysfunctional.

Trachoma, a bacterial infection of the eye, and **pemphigoid**, an autoimmune disorder, are other conditions that attack the mucous membranes and lead to scarring and altered function of the tear production mechanism.

If this catalogue of diseases and conditions you've just read through seems scary, I can only assure you there's no need to be frightened. Chances are that if you have one of the serious diseases or conditions mentioned, you already know it. And the likelihood is that if you have dry eye, the cause is a simple one and the determination of an effective treatment easy to achieve.

Still, knowing these myriad possible causes of the disorder—and there are many more—will better equip you to work with your eye doctor to determine whether you have dry eye, why you have it, and how best to treat it.

3

WHAT TO EXPECT IN THE DOCTOR'S OFFICE

There is no cure for dry eye. But its irritations can most certainly be alleviated and its effects most certainly treated—both for the comfort of the patient and to staunch any further erosion of the health of the ocular surface.

It's important at the outset to clarify the difference between eye care professionals. You may be appropriately treated by an optometrist or an ophthalmologist. Optometrists are trained to examine the eyes, identify and diagnose problems, and prescribe contact lenses and eyeglasses. Optometrists are not medical doctors and may not perform surgery or, in some states, prescribe oral medications, but they may be very skilled in treating dry eye. An opththalmologist is a medical doctor who specializes in the eye—its function, its pathology, and its treatment, including surgery, drugs, or any other eye procedure. Some opthalmologists specialize in diseases of the cornea and the outside of the eye and are particularly experienced in treating dry eye. Opticians make and dispense eyeglasses and are not eye care professionals.

Diagnosis is of course the first step toward determining the treatment that can achieve both those goals. Finding out whether a patient has dry eye, the source of his or her dry eye, and the effect the disorder may be having on the ocular surface is essential to identifying the right therapy that will bring the patient relief and restore the health of the eye as much as possible.

And diagnosis is much like detective work. It's a matter of gathering evidence, sifting clues, and eliminating what doesn't "fit" until you're left with a positive conclusion. We doctors use a number of tools for that: observation, history, examination, and scientific testing employing a range of different technologies. You should expect your eye doctor to use any or all of the tools at his or her disposal when you show up for your appointment complaining of dry eye symptoms.

Observation and the 'History'

The first thing I do when I see a patient is observe. I can learn a lot about a patient's overall eye health and vision just by noting how and how often the person blinks, the anatomy of his or her facial structure, the condition of the eyes and of the surrounding skin and muscles, even posture and the way patients carry themselves. Like most doctors, I've found out some important information before I've asked a single question.

The questioning itself is key. The term of art is "taking a history," and in doing so, your doctor really puts together a profile of your health in general and gleans information, not readily observable, that may explain a lot about the particular ailment you're complaining about—and about what to look for if you're not complaining at all.

You can help, too. The more information patients can bring to the doctor's office, the more efficient and ultimately the more effective the physician's observation, examination, and testing will be.

Here's a questionnaire that can make a significant difference when your eye doctor starts taking a history. My suggestion? Fill it out and take this book with you to your next eye exam. Your doctor will thank you for it.

Question	Your Answer
Why are you seeking medical care for your eyes?	
What's sending you to the eye doctor's office?	
What symptom bothers you the most?	
Put it this way: if you could ask your eye doctor to fix only one thing, what would it be?	
When did you last feel perfectly healthy in your eyes?	
Is one eye worse than the other?	
What makes your eyes feel worse?	
What makes your eyes feel better?	
Is there a difference in your level of discomfort between night and day?	
Have you traveled recently? Where?	
Was your travel to a very different climate and environment?	
How did you feel there?	
Does eating certain foods make your eyes feel worse or better?	
What medicines do you take — including vitamins, supplements, and over-the-counter treatments both oral and topical?	
Have you ever had surgery? For what condition?	
Have you ever had a cosmetic procedure on your eyes or face?	
Do you wear contact lenses? Soft or hard? Overnight?	

Question	Your Answer
How many hours per day and days per week do you typically keep your lenses in?	
Have you recently begun to find your lenses uncomfortable?	
Do you sleep on your stomach, back, or side?	
Do you get up in the night? How frequently?	
On first awakening, how do your eyes feel?	
Do you have any food, medicine, or environmental allergies?	
What is your occupation? What's the substance of your job — that is, what do you actually do all day?	
How would you describe your workplace environment?	

Examination with a Slit Lamp

After taking your history, your eye doctor will examine your eyes through a slit lamp. The slit lamp is what the eye doctor looks through when you are seated with your chin settled into the chin rest and your forehead supported. It looks like a microscope but is basically a very high-intensity light and a magnifier so that the doctor can examine the structure of your eye inside and out.

Looking through the slit lamp, your eye doctor can get a good look at your eyelid margin. He or she can check for meibomian gland dysfunction and can ascertain if you have blepharitis, an inflammation of the eyelid margin. You might feel the doctor apply light pressure to the eyelid glands to see if something comes out, and to check whether what emerges is a clear liquid or a viscous discharge that might be yellowish, milky, or greenish in color.

In addition, the doctor may ask you to close your eyes; then, looking upward, he or she may be able to determine if you have lagophthalmos or if your eyelid closes fully. In these ways, it may be possible for the eye doctor to determine whether or not you have dry eye just by looking through the slit lamp.

Other Tests for Dry Eye

There are a number of different tests for dry eye, as well as tests that help determine the cause of the dry eye and measure its extent and impact. However, with one exception, the tests tend to be minimally reliable—so minimally that many opthalmologists have stopped using the tests. Since the test methodologies are variable and not reproducible, a negative result may not be conclusive, so the doctor will likely perform more than one test for dry eye—or even an array of tests of varying levels of sophistication. Consistent negatives across a range of these tests mean you do not have dry eye, but a mix of results indicates a need for further testing—or will lead to a diagnosis of dry eye.

TNT: DR. LATKANY'S DRY EYE TEST

No, my TNT is not an explosive, although I like to think that the Tear Normalization Test I've devised—the TNT—will ignite something of a revolution in the way ophthalmologists test for dry eye. I presented the TNT and my findings about its efficacy at a national conference of ophthalmologists in 2005. At the time, it was honored for the innovativeness of the concept and research; since then, more and more doctors have made it the standard test for their patients. Among other benefits, the TNT is the one exception to the minimal-reliability problem with most dry eye tests; its results have proven to be conclusive.

What's more, you can easily perform a version of the test at home. Of course, the home version does not yield a scientific result; it does not offer the level of precision an ophthalmologic technician or doctor can obtain in the examination room, under controlled conditions, with measurements carefully calculated. But it can provide a reasonable indication that you do or do not have dry eye.

All you need for the home test are the vision test on page 216, a small bottle of artificial tear drops—Allergan's Refresh Plus or Bausch & Lomb's Moisture Eyes or TheraTears will all do nicely—and a minute or two of time. (Make sure the drops are non-viscous, typically described as "for mild dry eyes;" anything thicker can actually blur your vision. If you like, you can use the finger test for viscosity; see the next chapter.) Stand the inside cover of the book/vision test card on a table or shelf, and keep stepping back until the top line of letters is just blurry enough that you can't really read the letters. Now put one or two drops of the artificial tears in each eye—try not to blink as you do this, or you might blink the tear away—and then look again at that blurry line of letters. If you can see the line clearly even for a split second, you probably have dry eye.

If that's the case, what has happened is that the moisture of the drops has normalized your tear film, and that has improved your visual acuity. But the improvement is temporary, lasting only for a few seconds up to perhaps a minute or so. Once the effects of the drops have worn off, the line of letters will again seem blurred.

In the doctor's office, the TNT will be performed only slightly differently. Your eye doctor—or a technician—will first check your vision in each eye by asking you to read lines of letters on a visual acuity chart with first one eye, then the other. Those results will be recorded, then artificial tear drops will be applied, and the doctor or technician will ask you again to read the highest line of letters you could not read before. Your responses will be measured and again recorded, providing a vision acuity benchmark for your medical chart.

Whether in the doctor's office or at home, however, the TNT is a reliable test: if your vision improves temporarily with the artificial tears, the likely permanent reality is that you have dry eye.

TESTING WITH DYE

Fluorescein is a yellow-orange dye routinely used for tracking problems in the ocular surface. One of the most common uses of fluorescein is a test for your tear break-up time—that is, for how long it takes for a break in the tear film to appear. The doctor or technician will put a small amount of the dye in your eye and ask you to blink. The blinking spreads the dye around the ocular surface. Then, looking through the slit lamp and using a blue light, the doctor or technician will literally count the seconds till the tear film breaks up. Anything under

10 seconds is considered abnormal and suggests that the patient has dry eye because of an unstable tear film.

That's important to know if, for example, your job requires you to sit in front of a computer all day. If so, and if you have a low tear break-up time, the chances are good that your tear film's defense wall is not as formidable as it should be. Bottom line? Your eye health is endangered, and symptoms of dryness will most likely become apparent soon.

Actually, a new methodology now makes it possible for eye doctors to check for tear break-up without the dye, so patients can now learn about the stability of their tear film without having to look at the world through fluorescein's yellow-orange "filter."

But fluorescein is needed for another test—the clearance test. In this test, after the dye has been applied, the doctor or technician dabs the eye with a small piece of filter paper. If the paper picks up the orange dye, it means that the fluorescein has not "cleared" the eye fast enough. It's still there on the ocular surface—and that typically means that the patient exhibits the symptoms of dry eye; the eye is simply not washing itself fast enough. In fact, the failure to clear is a result of inflammation, and as a consequence, the inflammatory agents remain on the surface of the eye, exacerbating the condition even further.

Fluorescein isn't the only dye used to test the tear film, although its particular property—it pools in a break or hole in the tear film—makes it especially useful for identifying gaps in the ocular surface, which appear green when examined with the blue light of the slit lamp. Two other dyes, one red and one green, are also used. Rose Bengal dye, the red one, and lissamine, which is green, both stain areas that are unhealthy—areas of dead cells perhaps, or of cells that are losing their protective capabilities. Both these dyes can detect problems that fluorescein misses, so it is not unusual for a doctor to apply more than one dye. Patients who have undergone such tests typically leave the doctor's office with eyes an odd color combination of red, green, and yellow—and they may maintain this scary look for upwards of half an hour. Don't worry; you'll soon be back to normal.

One cautionary note: some people are allergic to dyes. If you know you have such an allergy, alert your eye doctor before any drops are placed in your eyes.

MEASURING TEARS

One of the most common eye exams is the Schirmer test, which measures the quantity of tears that the eye produces in a specified period of time. A piece of filter paper is placed onto your lower eyelid and positioned between the eyelid and the eyeball. It stays there, with the patient's eyes closed, for about five minutes. When it's removed, it shows a measurement of the amount of moisture that has been produced. Obviously, a low moisture count is a signal of possible dry eye.

Another test, which achieves a very objective assessment of the tear film, measures its osmolarity—that is, the ability of the tear film to be diffused between membranes. Remember your high-school chemistry class when you learned how water on one side of a membrane will diffuse to salt on the other side of the membrane, moving from an area of high water concentration to an area of lower water concentration? The same principle is at work here; the tear film, being mostly water, should diffuse easily. To find out just how easily, the doctor or technician captures a small sample of your tear, and a machine then measures its concentration and therefore its

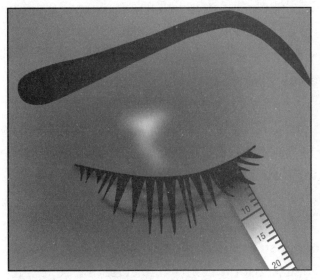

Figure 5: *The Schirmer test measures tear production with a piece of filter paper*

osmotic capability. Higher osmolarity means a less watery tear film—i.e., a tear film that does not diffuse easily. That, in turn, makes it more likely that you have dry eye.

Yet another test—a highly sophisticated one—can measure the proteins found in the tear film. As the quantity and concentration of proteins tend to decrease with age, a lowered number and concentration either signal or anticipate a patient's dry eye.

TESTING FOR SPECIFIC CAUSES

Other tests evaluate specific conditions of dry eye and help doctors determine the first cause or origin of the disorder. One such test—it sounds more unpleasant than it is—is to stick a cotton swab up the nose in order to stimulate a tearing reflex. If nothing happens—if the reflex does not go off and no tears are produced—the patient may well have Sjögren's syndrome, since Sjögren's patients have no reflex tears. By contrast, if the test stimulates the tear reflex, the patient almost certainly does not have Sjögren's syndrome.

An ocular surface sensitivity test can discover dry eye in patients who are asymptomatic—that is, who report no symptoms of the disorder. The doctor might use a fine cotton thread or strand of nylon filament to touch various parts of the eye. Most normal patients will feel the touches; remember, after all, that the cornea has the highest concentration of nerve fiber endings of any structure in the body. But people whose capability for neural sensation has been affected (diabetics, herpes sufferers, and people who have had a LASIK eye procedure) may not respond as noticeably to the touches. This means they also don't sense when their eyes are dry. Their eyes are therefore not sending dryness messages to the brain, and the brain is therefore not being stimulated to send messages to the muscles telling them to blink and to start secreting tears. So even if these patients don't complain of dry eye symptoms, this sensitivity test will give a pretty good indication of why an asymptomatic dry eye patient is asymptomatic. It's important to treat such patients aggressively precisely because they cannot detect their own symptoms and need just that much more protection of the ocular surface than patients who feel and complain of the disorder.

As for determining which disease or condition may be the antecedent of dry eye, that mostly requires blood tests that look for serum antibodies that will mark the presence of Sjögren's syndrome or rheumatoid arthritis or lupus or the like. The four that are typically performed are ANA, SS-A, SS-B, and RF; more than half of Sjögren's syndrome sufferers get positive results in these tests—not a resounding indication of the syndrome but certainly one of the criteria for diagnosis. Your eye doctor can order these tests, or he or she may refer you to a specialist like a rheumatologist or to your primary care physician for a history and complete physical as well as the tests.

Another test can detect the number of goblet cells on the ocular surface. The test requires rubbing a nitrocellulose membrane across the whites of the eyes; then, through impression cytology, researchers can literally count the goblet cells on the surface. If there is an insufficient number of goblet cells, your doctor can be pretty sure you have dry eye; he or she will also know that the cause is a problem in the mucous layer of the tear film, the layer the goblet cells produce.

Once the tests have been completed and the results are in, and once you and your doctor have worked together to create a profile of your eye health, it's time to look to the range of treatments available for dry eye—and to identify the one that will work for you.

4

What Over-the-Counter Treatments Can—and Can't—Do to Help

Walk into any good-sized drugstore these days, find your way to the aisle marked "eye care," and you'll confront a dizzying array of product options. Here are tears, gels, sprays, and ointments aimed at every possible variant of eye distress: dryness, irritation, redness, allergies, pinkeye, eyes that stare at a computer all day, eyes that don't close fully at night, eyes that are slightly itchy, moderately itchy, very itchy, and very, very itchy. There are clear solutions, solutions in a range of viscosity levels, gels and ointments that promise to coat the eye for long-lasting relief, and "botanical" oils and unguents that claim to alleviate your distress naturally. A company called Nature's Tears has even come up with a mist that you spray at your eyes—highly useful for those who recoil from using an eye dropper and/or who like the idea of a refreshing mist vaporizing toward them like a gentle rain.

The profusion of these over-the-counter treatments can be downright confusing. And in fact, studies of buying behavior show that what typically guides people's behavior when it comes to these products are price and advertising—they either choose the cheapest of the items on display or the ones that are most heavily advertised. Yet the products keep rolling down the pipeline, as if the manufacturers had gotten the message that one size of eye care solution does not fit all.

That is certainly true. Within the category of dry eye disorder alone, as we have seen, one can find various types of irritation and differing needs for relief. The companies that manufacture these increasingly numerous over-the-counter eye treatments are to be commended for continuing to research and develop a range of products to meet a range of eye care needs arising from a range of conditions. But what goes unspoken amid all the claims and very real benefits of these over-the-counter treatments is this single fact: none of them get at the source of the problem. They are all palliatives; they offer only temporary relief from the eye distress you are feeling.

That is why it is absolutely essential that these over-the-counter treatments are used appropriately—carefully, sparingly, with an understanding of their limitations, and with knowledge about what's in them.

Let's just take one example to illustrate why: the example of that proverbial person who works in front of a computer all day—we'll call her Mary. By lunchtime, Mary's eyes feel as dry and irritated as sandpaper in the desert, and she is desperate for some kind of relief. So on her lunch hour, she trots over to the nearest discount drugstore and scans the shelves. Naturally, she looks for a treatment that is clear, not viscous. Mary's job depends on sharp eyesight, and thickly gooey artificial tears, which offer a nicely soothing coating over the ocular surface, will blur her vision. On the other hand, a non-viscous solution, precisely because it doesn't coat the eye for long, will need to be applied more frequently. That means time taken from the job as Mary continually heads for the ladies' room to irrigate her eyes yet again. It also means a fair piece of change spent on artificial tears that need to be replaced with unremitting frequency.

And even if Mary finds just the right artificial tears—ones that alleviate her distress without affecting her vision too badly and that only need to be applied perhaps once an hour—she still hasn't done anything about what's wrong with her eyes.

That's because, as you now know, what's wrong with Mary's eyes is a deficient quantity or quality of tears. Certainly, as we've learned, if she puts some aqueous liquid into her eyes, she will feel relief. The liquid will coat the eye, serving as artificial tears, but once it has evaporated, she'll be right back where she started—with a deficient quantity or quality of tears.

In a study I authored on the impact of artificial tears on vision, we found that non-viscous drops improve the vision wonderfully—for up to four and a half minutes. It's likely that that's how long the relief from irritation lasts as well, although such a measurement is highly individual and highly subjective. The point is that the impact lasts only as long as the solution remains in the eye. As the study made clear, once the artificial tears had evaporated or been blinked away, there was no lasting palliative influence—because there had been no fundamental therapeutic action.

That's why it's so important to know what's in the artificial tears that poor Mary keeps squirting into her eyes—especially because she has found after a while that she needs the drops more and more frequently. What exactly is this stuff? Could it be causing side effects? And why does she need it more frequently and not less frequently? Could it be exacerbating the problem rather than helping it? All good questions; they should be answered before anyone introduces anything into their eyes.

Does this mean that traditional over-the-counter treatments are useless? Not at all. In fact, they perform an important function, for there are very often times when palliative relief is exactly what is needed. That is precisely why these products have traditionally constituted the first line of treatment for eye complaints. Your eyes bother you, and you go to the drugstore and buy some drops. Or, at your annual eye exam, you tell your eye doctor that your eyes feel dry, and you are offered a sample of the latest artificial tear product and told to come back in a year. You get home, pop in the drops, and—aaaah!—the relief is immediate.

It is only with time, as you keep using the drops, and as you find you must use them more and more frequently, that the product proves to be insufficient. You reach a point of diminishing returns, and you are at best back at square one and at worst deteriorating.

The answer, therefore, if you are going to use these over-the-counter products effectively and successfully, is to know what they can and cannot do—their capabilities and their limits—and to understand that they are relief for your irritation, not remedies for your dry eye disorder.

Think of these traditional over-the-counter treatments in terms of four basic categories:

- Artificial tears, gels, sprays, and ointments
- Redness removers
- Contact lens cleaning and wetting solutions
- Homeopathic or "natural" treatments

Let's take them one at a time.

Artificial Tears

Artificial tears are probably the most common over-the-counter treatments used for dry eye—whether you buy them for yourself or your eye doctor recommends them. Officially known as hydrogels, they are simply compounds that try to mimic the natural tear film; they act as a "replacement" for your own deficient tears and help you hold out against the too-rapid evaporation taking place as a result of some deeper cause.

It's unlikely, in my view, that the pharmaceutical companies will achieve the actual equivalent of human tear film any time soon. Nature's tear film is too complex, and the synergy of the composition is quite likely matchless. But researchers keep working at it, and they continue to come up with new combinations of ingredients that in one way or another approximate aspects of a healthy human tear film.

These over-the-counter artificial tear products come in varying viscosities. From the least viscous to the most viscous, you will see them labeled as plain or mild, long-lasting or moderate, severe or highly viscous or liquid gel, and finally as ointment, the most viscous of all. Viscosity in these solutions is like viscosity in any fluid; it's a measure of how "thick" the fluid is and how resistant it is to flowing or being poured. The more viscous the tears—the gummier they are—the better they will coat the ocular surface, the more symptoms they will attempt to address, and the longer their palliative effect will last. But of course, the more viscous tears will also blur the vision more, and that blur can itself be an annoyance. A product labeled a "liquid gel" will cover a number of annoyances and irritations and will last at least an hour and maybe two. But the initial blur it produces can be as vexing as a foreign object in the eye, although the blur will fade as the drops dissipate, and by the time they are gone from the eye, the blur will be gone as well.

The Finger Test for Viscosity

You can see for yourself how viscosity works by performing a simple test. Put a drop of your artificial tears on your index finger and rub it with your thumb. If it feels like water, it has low viscosity; if it feels like cooking oil, it has high viscosity; if it feels somewhere in between the two, you can calibrate for yourself how viscous it is.

But a great many brands of over-the-counter artificial tears have another ingredient in addition to their tear-film-like compound—namely, a preservative—and sometimes, that can be a problem, as a patient I'll call Linda found out.

The outward sign of Linda's problem was obvious: at first glance, I could see that her lower eyelids were red, especially in the corners closest to her nose; in fact, the redness continued on the skin alongside both sides of her nose. Linda was 45, had had little trouble with her eyes for most of her life, and admitted that her eyes were killing her. They were red, itchy, and dry, and everything she had tried had helped only temporarily. By the time she came to see me, she was using artificial tears every 15 minutes and, in her words, "going absolutely crazy."

She came to our appointment carrying a list of all the solutions she had tried. Linda's list was a roll call of just about every available over-the-counter artificial teardrop; the most recent one contained a commonly used preservative, benzalkonium chloride. And that was the tip-off that told all.

I understood from Linda's list that she had a baseline level of dryness. What was making it worse, however, was her self-medicating with artificial teardrops. She had been doing so for a couple of years; she had been using the tears with benzalkonium chloride for a couple of months. Now, she was experiencing an allergic reaction that was outlined by the redness on her face. Think about it. If you've ever put too big a drop or too many drops in your eyes, you've felt and seen the excess typically flowing down from the inside corner alongside the nose. That was where Linda's skin was the reddest—following the trail of her excess tears down her face.

It was time for Linda to stop using drops altogether. Instead, I prescribed a mild steroid salve to calm the itchiness and told her to report back in 10 days. When she did, the redness was gone. The upshot was that we were back at square one—back at the baseline level of dryness, the original cause of Linda's distress. With an end to the self-treatment that had made her distress worse, we could start treating the underlying problem. And that's exactly what we did.

Most eye drops do contain preservatives—either the one that caused Linda's problem or any of a range of others. The preservatives are there for protection; they reduce the possibility that bacteria might thrive in the closed environment of the bottle. The problem is that the preservatives promote inflammatory changes that could disrupt the tear film. What's more, they can very often be an allergen to very many people. In fact, the preservative that bothered Linda, benzalkonium chloride, perhaps the most commonly used preservative in artificial tears—it's found in 5 of the top 25 sellers in the country—has

Allergy Alert!

If you tend to have allergies, look out for these ingredients often used as preservatives in artificial tears. Check the label carefully for: polyquad, sodium perborate, purite, sodium silver chloride, sorbic acid, chlorobutanol, polyquaternium-1, polyhexamethylene biguanide (PHMB), Dissipate, thimerosal, and of course benzalkonium chloride.

been shown to cause highly allergic reactions in some people. That's why it's important to know what preservative is in the tears you take and to consult with your physician about its allergic potential, if any.

But there is another problem with the preservatives in so many artificial tears. Over time, their effect can exacerbate dry eye symptoms and even potentially harm the ocular surface. If, as often happens, you find yourself using the drops more and more frequently as their impact grows less and less effective—the point of diminishing returns—you may be simply flooding your eyes with chemicals that eventually erode your eye health.

But of course, there are cases where medications with preservatives may be all that's available—or may simply be necessary for another ailment or condition. Susan offers a case in point.

At age 84, Susan was diabetic, suffered from glaucoma, and was beginning to have troubles with short-term memory. She also had eyes that were extremely red and irritated, which is why her glaucoma specialist referred her to me.

Susan arrived for the appointment carrying a veritable sack of what she called her "eye medicines." She pulled them out, one by one, and lined them up on the table between us: some 15 bottles of different medications, recommended or suggested or prescribed by some six different doctors. The problem was that Susan simply could not keep straight which medicine was suggested for which condition. Since she didn't want to take any chances that she would be missing the one she needed, her solution was to take them all.

My first thought was that Susan's eyes were irritated

because there was simply too much medicine in them—and probably too many preservatives in the medicines. I consulted with her glaucoma specialist, and we were able to narrow down the 15 medications to 3 essential glaucoma treatments. But to try to reduce the amount of preservatives in Susan's very irritated eyes, I made a call to Leiter's Pharmacy in San Jose, California, specialists in non-preservative medications for the eyes—and for the rest of the body. Sure enough, I was able to find a glaucoma treatment that was preservative-free. The upshot for Susan? She needed no dry eye treatment at all; she simply needed to stop delivering highly allergenic preservatives into her eye.

Susan's case presents an object lesson for patients taking needed medications for such other eye conditions as glaucoma. It's important to be aware that many of these medications do contain preservatives. If you're taking such drops and have symptoms of dry eye, you need to consult with your eye doctor concerning your options.

PRESERVATIVE-FREE DROPS

A much better choice in artificial tears is preservative-free drops. These typically come in sealed single-use vials; uncap the vial, apply the drops, dispose of the vial. Although it may be somewhat bothersome to have to carry these vials around, and although the drops are certainly more expensive than those with preservative, the cost in inconvenience and money is more than repaid by the fact that you're not putting potentially harmful chemicals into your eyes.

The Cost vs. Waste Issue

The prices for artificial tears range from about $5 to $25 depending on the size of the package, which typically contains from 5 to 30 milliliters of product. The cost seems reasonable enough—if buyers get the full value from their purchase. All too often, they may not.

Even a drop at a time, the waste can be substantial. The bottles tend to dispense fairly large drops, yet the eye can typically only take half an eye drop. It means that much of what you apply can end up rolling down your cheek. Or if you have trouble applying the drops and you miss a few drops each time you try, the bottle may empty sooner rather than later.

What's more, these bottles are small, easy to lose, and very easy to leave uncapped, which may lead to the contents becoming infected—a total waste.

Most wasteful of all is if the individual becomes dissatisfied because the drops have ceased to work. At that point, of course, even $5 is too expensive.

I'm a big fan of preservative-free artificial tears, and when I recommend them to my patients, as I often do, I suggest they refrigerate the tears. Chilled drops feel wonderful on an irritated eye, and you can tell with absolute certainty that the drop has hit the eye, so you tend not to waste drops down your cheek. What's more, the effect lasts longer when the drops are chilled, and the chill adds a sterility factor. My claims about the benefits of refrigerating artificial tears have been confirmed by a study reported in 1997; it found that cold artificial tears reduce inflammation and corneal and conjunctival sensation—that is, they're more comfortable to patients.

In fact, so many of my patients have been converted to the idea of chilled tears that I developed an eye drop bottle carrier for them—a small, insulated, pocket-sized pouch with enough room for a few bottles. The carrier keeps the tears separate and isolated so the bottles don't get lost in the jumble of a typical purse or briefcase, and it will keep the tears feeling cold for several hours. But I've also made an ice pack to fit the carrier, and this means that the tears stay delightfully chilled all day long. You just have to remember to put the ice pack in the freezer at home each night to get that longer-lasting effect.

My aim in creating the carrier was simply to make it easier for patients to use the drops regularly, for failure of compliance with a doctor's recommendation can be a real impediment to getting the relief patients seek. The convenience of the carrier means the tears can be on hand at all times, and having them on hand makes it easy to apply them.

OINTMENTS

Ophthalmic ointments may also come in a preservative-free version, although many do contain preservatives. They also have a higher concentration of the tear-like compound, which accounts for some of their higher viscosity, and they may also contain mineral oil and petrolatum. One of the major selling points of the ointments, which come in varying viscosities, is that they are longer-lasting than less viscous solutions. Two hours or more is a not uncommon duration for the palliative impact of ointments, although vision may be blurry for a good portion of that time.

I often recommend ointments to my patients at night when vision is not so terribly important. Refresh PM from Allergan, Lacrilube, and Genteal Gel from Novartis are among those preferred by my patients. For lagophthalmos sufferers, in particular, ointments can be extremely effective. To be sure, patients often wake with a film over their vision, but it dissipates in due course. In the meantime, their eyes have been coated and protected all night long.

But whether ointment or gel or drops, the very variety of artificial tears—and the variety of the compounds and preservatives within them—means that finding the one that's right for you could be a process of trial and error. To narrow your focus, it's best to know what's wrong with your eyes, know your allergies, and talk to both your eye doctor and your primary care physician. Thus armed, you'll be ready to face that dizzying array of products, and you'll have a goal in mind as you try to find the artificial tear that is right for you. And if you can, make it one without preservatives.

Redness Removers

Almost everybody has tried redness-removing eye drops. Visine, which coined the phrase, "Get the Red Out," is a household name—probably the only one among eye care solutions. Visine works. So do other redness removers. They all get the red out.

Fresh from the Pipeline...

As of this writing, research and development in both the content of artificial tears and their packaging offer some exciting new possibilities. A new sub-category of preservative-free tears is now available in the form of a disappearing preservative—it goes away the moment the drops make contact with the eye—and in a new bottle from Pfizer that uses an ingenious inner chamber and air-lock technology to maintain the sterility of the contents without a preservative.

Other research has focused on approximating tear film more precisely and tailoring the artificial tears to specific tear film deficiencies. **TheraTears** from Advanced Vision Research, for example, closely approximates the electrolytes of natural tears and thus helps restore the electrolyte balance of the tear film.

Systane, a new drop from Alcon, contains the compound HP-guar which has a unique property: it acquiers a gel-like consistency in the eye and binds into a protective coating. It lasts quite a while despite fairly low viscosity, offering only a slight blur that dissipates quickly. Alcon now offers a gel variety of Systane in a bottle; it's good to see that this product is preservative-free—so important in a product used so frequently.

From Alimera Sciences comes **Soothe**. It's basically a lipid—with a preservative, PHMB—and it is targeted at patients with a deteriorated or inefficient oily layer. It contains a component called Restoryl, a combination of oil and water, which beefs up both the oily or lipid layer and the aqueous layer to create a more stable tear film. Though Soothe hasn't been around long enough for us to know all it can do, it is evidence, along with Systane and others, that over-the-counter artificial tears are just getting better, more focused, and more effective.

They do it by temporarily constricting the blood vessels that have become dilated, inflamed, and angry-looking in your eyes. They are vasoconstricting agents, and they make the vessels less apparent—and the whites of your eyes correspondingly less red. Vasoconstricting agents are highly effective, therefore, at addressing a symptom, but they in no way address the problem causing the symptom.

There are some dangers in using these agents. First, they contain preservatives which can cause allergic reactions. Second, they may produce harmful side effects—including glaucoma. Third, they're subject to a rebound effect—that is, the more you use a vasoconstrictor, the shorter the time it lasts, and the rebound from its action makes your eyes redder than they were before. Finally, because vasoconstrictors are convenient and inexpensive, users run the risk of overdoing their application to the point of self-medication.

There's a definite place for vasoconstrictors. Perhaps you have an important business engagement, or a very important dinner date, or it's your turn to get your photo taken for the company magazine, or you've simply had a bad day and your eyes are bloodshot. Drop in a vasoconstrictor and you'll look and feel better long enough to meet the momentary need.

But do use these agents sparingly, and see your doctor if you find your usage becoming more frequent than twice a month.

Contact Lens Solutions

Contact lens wearers who suffer from dry eye must add an additional factor—the lenses themselves—to their equation of concern in choosing eye care treatments. The issue is the same—know what you're putting in your eyes—but it is complicated by the presence of the lenses, whether they're soft or gas-permeable, and by the type of cleansing, conditioning, and wetting solutions the lens wearers choose to use.

The pharmaceutical companies market a number of dryness drops directly to contact lens wearers on the theory that they constitute a distinctive "niche" market. Indeed they do, although in some cases the content of the drops may not be very different from the compounds marketed to the general public. What really distinguishes lens wearers is this extra level of caution they need to add to their choice of dryness solutions, as Ted's story makes clear.

Ted was 25 and had worn soft contact lenses for seven years. In the last year, however, he had found it increasingly difficult to tolerate wearing his lenses for more than a few hours at a time. His eyes would feel dry, irritated, and scratchy until he finally had to take the lenses out, clean them again, feed artificial tears into his eyes for relief, then pop the lenses back in—only to go through the whole process all over again a few hours later.

Ted had also had three cases of what he described, when he came to see me, as pinkeye. "Why do I keep getting these colds in my eyes?" Ted asked, "and why am I having such trouble wearing my lenses?"

Three cases of conjunctivitis—what Ted called pinkeye—in a year seemed excessive; the pinkness Ted ascribed to colds had to be due to something else. The "something else" became clear the moment I looked under Ted's eyelids, where I could see a smattering of good-sized bumps, called papillae, right on the underside of his eyelid. These papillae are not uncommon in wearers of soft lenses, and because of their size—they are really quite substantial—the condition they represent is called Giant Papillary Conjunctivitis, or GPC. GPC is a severe allergic reaction that substantively decreases an individual's tolerance for wearing contact lenses—sometimes for months, sometimes forever.

The question was: what caused Ted's GPC? While the lenses themselves can generate the condition, they're not necessarily the only factor; dryness, for example, may be a contributing cause. And since Ted had had no problem tolerating his lenses until a year ago, it seemed likely that some event at that time had precipitated his problem. What happened a year ago? Had he changed his lenses?

"No," answered Ted.

"What about your solution?"

"Well, yes," he said, surprised at the recollection. "About a year ago, I changed the cleaning solution I use, and at the same time, I decided to buy wetting solution of that same brand."

"Why?" I asked. "What was the reason for the change?"

"No reason," Ted replied, "except that I moved, and the drug-store near my new apartment didn't carry my old brand."

The coincidence was too great to ignore. I recommended to Ted that he stop wearing his lenses altogether and that he throw away his cleaning and wetting solutions. Meanwhile, I pre-scribed a topical salve for the irritation. It took a little more than a month for Ted's case of GPC to clear up entirely; this made it seem most likely that his problem had been an allergic reaction to the new solution or wetting agent—or both. The issue then was to find a better way for Ted to wear and tolerate lenses as well as a solution that would give him relief from his dryness without causing an allergic reaction.

Today, Ted uses daily disposable lenses; with nothing to store or clean, there's little chance of bacterial intrusion. For the dry-ness, Ted relies on preservative-free wetting drops marketed especially to soft-lens wearers. He also follows the recommen-dation I make to all my patients who wear lenses: take a break. Wear your lenses five days a week, not seven—what I call the "contact lens holiday."

Not all contact lens wearers are allergic to the solutions they use, or to preservatives. But it's important for them to know that the solutions marketed to them may contain preservatives—like those used in eyedrops—and these could exacerbate their dryness.

Moreover, there are some drops that simply should not be used with lenses at all. Thickly viscous drops, for example, can be a particular problem with soft lenses—not just because they will blur the vision, but because the drops stick to the lenses. This can cause a build-up of proteins and possibly bacteria. And the last thing anyone wants is a situation in which you are introducing something unhealthy into your eyes each time you put in your lenses. Of course, lens wearers can use the viscous drops when their lenses are out of their eyes.

There are now also lenses that are made specifically for dry eye patients. Manufacturers are using new materials that are softer, and moister, and allow the eye to breathe a bit better. So if you're a lens wearer, think about switching, and talk to your eye doctor. But even if you do switch—and many of my patients have found great success with the new versions—don't wear your lenses non-stop. Cut down on the wear time, take breaks, give your eyes a chance to recover—and you'll be able to wear contact lenses safely and happily for life.

Homeopathic Treatments

Homeopathy is a venerable and well established "alternative" approach to healing. The idea behind homeopathy is a simple one: to introduce ingredients that stimulate a physiological reaction of the body's own healing mechanism. Of course, this is what a flu shot tries to do as well, but the active ingredients in homeopathic remedies are present in very small concentration and greatly diluted—just sufficient, according to homeopathic theory, to jump-start the immune system. Over-the-counter homeopathic products, the formulation and manufacture of which are regulated by the Food & Drug Administration, are widely available in mainstream as well as health-food stores. Many of my patients have reported extremely good results with

Similasan, one of the prominent favorites in this category, offering products for a range of eye irritations.

The idea behind homeopathy is certainly worthy, but the same rule applies to these dryness solutions as to the pharmaceutical brands: you need to know what's in them. Sometimes, it's all a matter of marketing; it sounds better to some people to think that they're using eyebright rather than aucubin, caffeic acid, ferulic acid, sterols, choline, and a volatile oil, which are the chemical components of eyebright. Certainly, reputable manufacturers like Similasan will list all ingredients faithfully, but it's up to you to beware of exactly what you're putting into your body.

A case in point is a patient I'll call Alice. A very elegant woman, Alice was a regular spa visitor and a devotee of natural ingredients. At 55 years of age, she had virtually no health worries; in fact, she had few worries of any kind. So when she suddenly developed some redness and puffiness around the face, she was keen to seek a natural remedy to deal with it, and she soon found just the thing: a homeopathic ointment that was advertised as being able to reduce puffiness. But just a few applications of the ointment caused a severe allergic reaction in Alice; the puffiness and redness actually increased. At that point, she consulted with an allergist who eventually was able to isolate one of the ingredients in the ointment—very healthy-sounding blue-green algae—as the allergen.

Four years later, Alice started feeling the discomforts of dry eye. As always, her first response had been to go to her local health-food store and browse the shelves for natural remedies.

The one she was using now, recommended by the health-store owner, was of private manufacture and had no label of ingredients; Alice had simply been told it would benefit dryness in the eyes. Yet after only a few uses, her eyes grew red and swollen. She brought the unlabeled ointment to her allergist who ran a check of the ingredients and found—not surprisingly-blue-green algae, the same allergen that had bothered her years before. It was at that point that Alice was referred to me; she is now undergoing dry eye treatments that steer clear of preservatives and other allergens—and certainly of blue-green algae.

The bottom line? Homeopathic remedies can be highly beneficial; in fact, I'm willing to guess they offer benefits we haven't yet guessed at. But no medication—and certainly nothing that you put in your eye—should be taken on faith. The claim of being "natural" or "botanical" is simply not sufficient. Without an ingredients list to consider, your doctor won't be able to know what the treatment addresses, how long you can take it, in what quantities, whether it has preservatives, what its side effects might be, and if it might cause something else to go wrong or exacerbate your dry eye over time.

By all means, shop for these homeopathic treatments, which can be wonderfully effective. But be sure you and your doctor know what's in them, and take as much care with their use as you would with pharmaceutical treatments.

All of these over-the-counter treatments—homeopathic or pharmaceutical, artificial tear or vasoconstrictor, liquid, gel, or ointment-can be effective when used appropriately. The key to doing so is to understand that any eye care treatment you buy in

a drugstore or health-food shop will offer only temporary benefits, not a long-term solution and certainly not a cure.

People sometimes assume that if a treatment doesn't require
a doctor's prescription, it can't hurt you. Yet as we've seen, indis-
criminate use of these eye care solutions—and using them to
self-medicate—can indeed hurt you with unwanted and harmful side effects, injury to your ocular surface and, in the worst
case, damaged vision.

But use these treatments sparingly, at the right time, in the right
way, and in consultation with your doctor, and their benefits can
be substantial.

PART TWO

RESTORING YOUR EYE HEALTH AT HOME

N ow that you know what can happen to cause or exacerbate dry eye, Part Two presents remedies and recommendations you can undertake on your own to restore the health of your eyes.

The truth is that the procedures and techniques outlined in the chapters of Part Two are sound medical advice for anyone and everyone, whether you're afflicted with dry eye or not. The recommendations about adjusting your environment, about lifestyle behaviors, and about possible changes in what you eat make good sense not just to prevent eye problems later on, but also to keep your eyes working at their best right now. And I routinely prescribe the Home Eye Spa procedures outlined in

Chapter 8 to all my patients—and would recommend them to anyone who cares about the health of their eyes.

But if you do have symptoms of dry eye, you may want to target the actions you undertake to restore the health of your eyes. So an important first step is to answer some key questions about your current habits and activities in four categories of activity. That's next.

5

YOUR DAILY ACTIVITIES

What do your commute to work, your television-watching preferences, and what you eat for breakfast have to do with the health of your eyes? The short answer is: a lot. As for the long answer, this chapter will help direct you to it.

It's simple: a solution to a problem—any solution to any problem—will work better if it addresses the core issue that specifically affects you. You wouldn't treat a strained muscle the same way you treat a broken bone, although both may cause you pain and limit your motion. Similarly, while dry eye is dry eye, it has a range of causes and may be affected by a range of factors. The better we can pinpoint the causes of and factors affecting your dry eye, the more pertinent the recommended treatment can be—and the quicker and more effective the benefit to you.

And daily life—the automatic habits and patterns of behavior you probably don't even think about anymore—can substantively affect the health of your eyes, the level of moistness on your ocular surface, and the chances for mitigating dryness.

That's why it's important to create a profile of your habits and behaviors at work, at home, eating and drinking, and at play. The answers you provide to the questions that follow will build that profile—and they can help direct you to the right set of recommendations for your particular dry eye condition.

I still recommend, however, that you read all of Part Two. There may be some causes or factors you haven't thought about that turn out to be in some way pertinent to your dry eye situation.

But for now, have a seat, find a pen or pencil, concentrate, and answer carefully the questions that follow:

WORK

Question	Yes	No
Do you commute to work by car?		
Do you use heat and/or air conditioning in your car?		
Does your work require that you spend time in front of the computer?		
Does your time in front of the computer exceed two hours a day?		
Do you work in a hermetically sealed building?		
Is your workstation or desk near an open window?		
Is your workstation or desk positioned in the path of currents of forced air from a heating/air-conditioning system?		
Do you travel on business?		
Does your business travel exceed three days per month?		
Do you frequently travel by plane?		

If you answered yes to five or more of these questions about work, pay particular attention to the environmental recommendations in Chapter 6.

HOME

Question	Yes	No
Do you spend more than two hours a day watching television?		
Is your television screen positioned higher than your head?		
Do you spend time at your home computer?		
Is your computer monitor positioned in such a way that you look upward at it?		
Is your favorite chair in the living room in the path of heated or cooled air from your heating or air-conditioning unit?		
Do you tend to cook with hot spices and other fragrant ingredients?		
Do you prefer baths to showers?		
Is your bed situated in such a way that currents of dry air from outside or from a heating or air-conditioning unit cross your face?		
Do you sleep fewer than seven hours a night?		

If you answered yes to four or more of the above questions, your eyes will benefit from the recommendations about lifestyle behavior in Chapter 7 as well as from the environmental adjustments outlined in Chapter 6.

EATING AND DRINKING

Question	Yes	No
Do you drink fewer than eight glasses of water a day?		
Do you drink coffee and/or tea?		
Do you like a cocktail before dinner or a nightcap before bed or a few beers on the weekend — i.e., are you a social drinker?		
Do you eat more steak than fish? More pizza than salad?		
Would you rather snack on potato chips than on an apple or a bunch of grapes?		
Do you walk right by the "organic food" counters in the market?		

If you answered yes to even two of the questions above, see the nutrition section in Chapter 7.

PLAY

Question	Yes	No
Do you play outdoor sports in your spare time?		
Do you engage in outdoor activities on week-ends-e.g., hiking, jogging, boating, skiing, etc.?		
Do you prefer dry climates to warm tropical locations for your vacations?		

Unless you answered no to all these questions, please focus on the lifestyle recommendations in Chapter 7.

No matter what answers you gave to any of the questionnaires, try the Home Eye Spa outlined in Chapter 8. Even if your eyes are perfectly healthy, you'll find that the Home Eye Spa is soothing and relaxing—and will help keep your eyes healthy.

6

YOUR ENVIRONMENT

Can normal, day-to-day doings in your own home cause or exacerbate dry eye? The answer is yes, as Sarah, a patient of mine who loves to cook, can explain.

Sarah was in her kitchen, whipping up one of her signature dishes, chicken Scarpariello with sausages. Her preferred recipe called for plenty of hot peppers, garlic, parsley, lemon, white wine, and other seasoning. But as Sarah browned the chicken and sautéed the sausages and tossed in the various herbs and other ingredients, and as the heat and the aromas of the different flavors began to fill the kitchen, her eyes suddenly started to burn and itch. This was serious pain, not a minor annoyance she could fix just by turning her head aside for a moment.

Sarah ran over to the window and, despite cold temperatures outside, flung it open; the blast of chilly air felt good at first, but it didn't alleviate her distress. She went into the living room and sat down in front of the fire to relax for a moment, but the dry warmth from the fireplace was no help at all. It wasn't until Sarah had closed her eyes for a good 30 seconds and put ice cubes over her eyelids, letting her eyes cool down and lubricate themselves once again, that the pain subsided. When she came to see me, her greatest concern, along with worry over the health of her eyes, was whether she would be able to cook in her kitchen again. She would, of course, once she began treatment for her rosacea-induced dry eye condition and learned how to adjust and deal with her cooking environment.

Benign as it seems—what could be more benign than your own kitchen?—your environment (the air, light, temperature, the objects you deal with) can contribute substantially to dry eye disorder and may counteract the beneficial effects of treatment. Even if you follow your doctor's recommendations to the letter, if you're in an inappropriate environment, you may still feel the symptoms of dry eye.

Ever been in a crowded elevator with someone wearing too much perfume? How about a smoky barroom? Ever walk past a candy store and get a strong whiff of rich chocolate—or walk past a spice store and take in a quick, harsh breath of curry or pepper? Have you ever found when you cook that, as happened to Sarah, the heat from the stove, filled with the intense aromas of oils and spices and other ingredients, irritated your eyes sufficiently that you had to turn away? Any of these "inappropriate" environmental situations can bring tears to your eyes. The perfume, the smoke, the rich or hot or spicy smells act as noxious stimulants that can irritate the ocular surface and promote an inflammatory response. Result? The tear reflex is jolted into action.

In a way, everyone experiences the symptoms of dry eye at some time in their lives, even if they are not diagnosed with dry eye disorder. Maybe you feel it in an airplane—a tightly sealed environment where dry, high-altitude air is pulled in from outside, then recycled around that small, enclosed space. You might be hiking in the desert. Or you might be visiting a friend who smokes, keeps his windows closed, and has invited you to watch the game on his wide-screen television tacked onto the wall a few feet over your head. Any of those environmental situations can contribute to dry eye, as we'll see, and you may find that by the end of the plane trip, or midway during the hike, or at half-time of the game that your eyes feel tired and irritated. Simply put, the conditions of your environment have overwhelmed the normal health of your tear film and dried out your eyes, setting off an inflammatory cascade, even if only temporarily.

For dry eye sufferers, of course, being in any such environment can be particularly uncomfortable—and can cause further deterioration of the ocular surface and of their overall eye health.

The good news, of course, is that we can make adjustments in our environment that will diminish its deleterious impact on dry eye disorder. We can also avoid environments that will exacerbate the dry eye. And where we don't control and cannot avoid the environment, we can still adjust our response to it in ways that mitigate its adverse effects.

At the Computer

Remember Mary, who sits in front of a computer all day and goes racing off to the discount drugstore on her lunch hour looking for artificial tears? Somebody has even given her problem a name—"computer vision syndrome." As more and more computers become essential to more and more jobs, it's likely that this syndrome will affect more and more people.

The syndrome has one very simple cause: staring. Today's high-powered computers are impressive pieces of equipment with lots of capabilities and an exciting graphical interface—and you just don't want to take your eyes off the screen. That's true whether you're in front of a computer because it's your job—tracking sales, which is what Mary does, or trading stocks, or writing—or because you're looking for entertainment, are surfing the internet, or keep your home records and communicate via email on the computer. Whatever the reason, when you use the computer, you stare, which means you don't blink. And when you don't blink, as you know, your tear film breaks up.

Sit in front of a computer for a while, perhaps to answer your email, and you can fairly easily tolerate the staring. But do it for two hours or so, and the symptoms of dry eye appear: your eyes feel tired, they burn, it's as if something is in them, they itch, and your vision starts to blur. For Mary, for stock traders who monitor the market in real-time, for air traffic controllers, even (as I can now testify) for writers, the long-term effect can be exhausting. I now know why authors at the end of a day of writing feel as physically tired as if they had run a marathon; their eyes have expended enormous effort to stay moist. The eyes are tired, and it makes the whole body feel weary.

Among other effects, such fatigue can lower productivity. When you're not feeling at your best, you tend not to think at your best. That can certainly have an impact on how well you do your job. If writers, and stock traders, and sales managers like Mary, could therefore adjust their computer-staring in small ways, they could keep their eyes from drying out, and I believe they will feel less tired as the day progresses. Feeling better, they will work better and more productively.

So what should they do to adjust their environment? The first thing to consider is the angle at which they stare at the computer monitor. Most people work at eye level with the screen. That means their eyes are fully open most of the time, exposing a good portion of the ocular surface. Some people actually set their monitors on platforms so that they look up at the screen. When they do that, they actually stretch their eyelids open even further, exposing the widest possible expanse of ocular surface to be "dried." It's the worst way to look at a computer screen.

A patient I'll call Joe takes the prize for the problems that can come from staring at a computer. A day trader, he spends eight hours at a stretch gazing upward at five separate color screens, all of them flashing and flickering at once on a platform high above his desk. Joe never wants to miss a single blip on any of the screens; he needs to be able to respond instantly to the tiniest shift in any market anywhere on earth. It's an exciting way to make a living, but it's also a breeding-ground for dry eye: Joe was both not blinking, so that he wouldn't miss a trick, and, because the screens were placed substantially above his head, he was forced to stretch his eyes open as wide as possible. The not-blinking served to break up his tear film, while his eyes expended maximum effort trying to coat the greatest possible amount of ocular surface with moisture. Needless to say, Joe's dry eye symptoms were just awful, and by the end of every trading day, he was utterly worn out—and therefore not doing his job with the kind of efficiency and sharp thinking it required.

The best way to look at a computer screen is down—at a small angle at least. That allows the upper eyelid to close a bit, exposing less of the ocular surface and enabling the eye to coat the surface effectively.

How do you adjust your environment so you're looking down at the computer monitor screen? That's easy: raise your chair and/or lower the position of the monitor. Joe did both—and it improved his dry eye and his energy level. He also took my advice and stood up periodically, using the opportunity to shake his arms and stretch his shoulders a bit. He was still staring at his five screens, but from an acute angle that allowed his eyelids to cover and thus coat much more of his ocular surface.

In addition to shifting the angle of your vision, take 10-second breaks. Turn away from the computer screen, close your eyes, move your eyeballs around underneath your closed lids to bathe and lubricate the eyes, count to 10, then open your eyes again. Do this twice an hour, and you'll mitigate your dry eye symptoms and feel far less tired at the end of a day.

I never could convince Joe that he could afford such breaks, but he promised instead to follow another recommendation and add a humidifier to his environment. It helped moisten the atmosphere—a big plus for the ever-watchful Joe. All you need is a small, portable unit. A half-gallon or gallon humidifier will do nicely. An easy-cleaning feature and an air purifier are pluses. Place the humidifier as close to your computer workstation as possible. As an addition to the twice-an-hour 10-second breaks, a humidifier can make a real difference in keeping your eyes moist. (If cost is an issue, try an open pan full of water on the radiator in winter.)

In Front of the Television

Some "home entertainment centers" have television screens that approximate the size of the screen down at the local multiplex. The new flat-panel televisions are not just huge; they're also pricey enough that no owner wants them anywhere near pets or small children. As a result, these flat panels are typically hung on the wall, well above eye level. As with the computer screen, looking up at a television stretches your eye open, exposing more of the ocular surface to be dried out.

Moreover, these monster screens are almost too much for the eye. There is so much going on and so much sheer territory to watch that you tend not to blink. After all, you don't want to miss anything.

Add to this situation the likelihood of warm or cold forced air, and even with a normal-sized screen, an evening of television-watching can be an incubator of dry eye symptoms.

Fortunately, your TV-watching is unquestionably within your control. Start by positioning the screen as low as you can—at least at eye level—and by positioning yourself out of the direct line of the air current. Take 10-second breaks to let your eyes lubricate themselves. During a commercial you don't want to watch anyway, try closing your eyes and just listening. And every now and again, stand up. Walk around. The television will still be there when you get back. Or TiVo it. If you do, you can then fast-forward through the ads and reduce the amount of time in front of the set-and thus of your continuous staring.

The Sleep Environment

Everyone wants to sleep well and long. And for anyone, creating a sleep environment that keeps the eyes moist is likely to result in a better, longer sleep. For most people, that goal is realized when they close their eyes and let the tear film's natural lubrication process kick in. But for people with lagophthalmos—that is, for people who sleep with their eyes slightly open—that doesn't happen.

As we learned earlier, researchers tell us that 5 to 10 percent of the population has lagophthalmos. I think the percentage is much higher. The percentage the researchers have measured comprises people with obvious lagophthalmos; their spouse or significant other or a friend or relative has reported to them that their eyes don't close completely during sleep. I believe that many more than 5 or 10 percent of Americans have obscure lagophthalmos, in which just a sliver of the ocular surface, too small for another person to notice, is exposed to the air. In a state—sleep—during which you are not blinking at all, even that sliver can be enough to dry out the eye completely, and that is why I believe that people who have no idea they have lagoph-thalmos complain of eye discharge in the morning and of eyes that are sticky, burning, and irritated on awakening. If you have those symptoms, check with your eye care professional, for only an expert can diagnose obscure lagopthalmos.

Moreover, people with either obvious or obscure lagophthalmos can inadvertently worsen their condition in a number of ways. People may take sleeping pills that indeed put them to sleep but also relax the muscle tone sufficiently that the eye doesn't remain closed; this worsens the lagophthalmos. Lots of people fall asleep with a hand on their face or their pillow scrunched up against their face; either situation could stretch the lids open even further, creating what is known as floppy eyelid syndrome.

But there are a number of steps lagophthalmos sufferers can take to help keep their eyes moist through the night. Ointments are available to keep the eyes wet, and some patients also tape their eyes shut. Even sleeping on your back, if possible, will help. And a humidifier positioned near the bed is always a good idea.

I also recommend the use of tranquileyes, from Eye Eco. This is a soft, flexible goggle—something like swim goggles, except that you cannot see through tranquileyes. Inside the goggle is a sponge you can soak in water; the goggle then forms an airtight seal around your eyes, creating a moist environment inside the goggle. The seal also prevents evaporation of either your natural tears or artificial tears. One model even has a small heating pad inside the goggle; this will loosen any clogged ducts.

All of these techniques will make the sleep environment more comfortable. That, in turn, will make the sleep better and longer, and it can help make the eyes feel better on awakening.

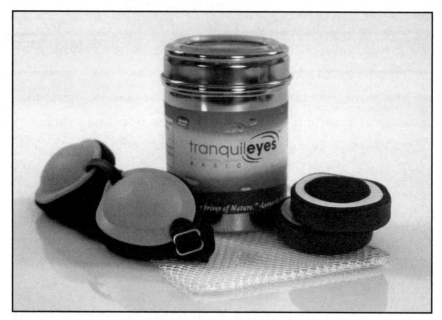

Figure 6: *tranquileyes goggles with sponge inserts*

Indoors

Most offices today—and many homes, too—are hermetically sealed environments which push forced-air heat at people during the winter months and blasts of cold air-conditioning at them during summer. Many buildings add ceiling fans that circulate the air further. One result is that people are almost always sitting in a current of air. Just as wet laundry on the line dries faster and better when there's a breeze, your tear film dries up quickly and uncomfortably when your eyes are constantly exposed to an air current.

Wherever you are, try to position yourself with the back of your head to the flow of the air. In other words, let the air current wash over you from behind, rather than meeting your eyes "head-on," so to say.

Humidity: It's All Relative

Many of today's home heating and cooling systems add a humidity component—with a separate humidistat on which you can both monitor the humidity in your home and set an optimum level, which a humidifying system then regulates. If you just happen to be building a new home or installing a new heating and cooling system, you might consider adding such a built-in humidifying option.

Until such systems are standard in housing, however, I recommend purchasing a home humidistat; it's like a digital thermometer, and is often combined with same, which measures the level of relative humidity in the immediate area. Actually, I recommend that you buy two—one for your bedroom, and one for whichever other room of the house you spend most of your time in. Then, become your own detective. Note when your eyes feel most and least comfortable, check the humidity for those levels of comfort and discomfort, and in time, you'll know precisely what level of relative humidity is ideal for you. That can be the benchmark around which you can adjust humidity levels—either by ratcheting up your home humidifier, opening a window, or even adjusting the heating and cooling thermostat. Here's a weekly chart that may help you with this monitoring:

Day	Room	Activity	Time	Comfort Rating (1–10)	Relative Humidity	Comments
Sunday						
Monday						
Tuesday						
Wednesday						
Thursday						
Friday						
Saturday						

Note where you were, what you were doing, and the time at each "reading." On a scale of 1 to 10, with 1 the least comfortable and 10 the most comfortable, rate how your eyes felt. Then note the humidity. Add any comments you think pertinent. At the end of the week, you should have a good idea of the ideal humidity for your eye comfort. Don't forget to repeat this exercise with every change of season.

You'll probably want to buy one or two home humidifiers to go along with your newfound knowledge so that you can more readily adjust the humidity to the ideal level. And you may also want to fiddle with the heating and cooling levels to fine-tune your comfort. But it's worth spending some time and effort on this so that you can be as comfortable as possible in your own home.

By the way, don't forget about houseplants. They humidify the air in addition to producing oxygen via photosynthesis. And of course, they bring beauty and pleasure into your home as well.

AIR PURITY

Melanie was 26 and couldn't figure out why her eyes were so red and itchy, although she noted that the redness and itchiness waxed and waned depending on what environment she was in. For a while, she thought the problem was the cat at her boyfriend's house, but her eyes were just as red and itchy at her house—and she had no cat.

So we tried an experiment. I asked if she could bear staying away from the boyfriend for several days. During that time, I suggested she clean everything in her house: all the bedding, all the rugs and carpets, all her clothing. The reason? Allergens— like those from Melanie's boyfriend's cat—can easily stick to your hair and clothing, then travel from there to your own living room and bedroom. True, there was no cat in Melanie's house, but there might as well have been. As it turned out, Melanie had brought the cat allergens home when she wore her boyfriend's sweatshirt. In her newly scrubbed and vacuumed home, Melanie felt fine; the minute she went over to his house, however, the redness and itchiness started up again.

It often takes that kind of investigation to find out exactly what is exacerbating your dry eye. But you can defend against such allergens—as well as against other impurities—by buying an air purifier. These fairly simple units, which are becoming increasingly affordable, literally pull the bad stuff out of the air and can make a real difference in reducing the risk that the atmosphere in your home or office may be irritating your eyes.

LOCATION LOCATION LOCATION

Finally, take a good look at exactly where you do most of your living—and check that particular environment to see if any adjustments should be made. Is your bed or the sofa where you read or watch TV directly in the path of an air current? If so, can you move either piece of furniture?

Is your bedroom or home office on the top floor of the house? Since heat rises, this is typically the warmest and driest level of the building, so perhaps you can think about relocating to a lower floor.

If you live in an apartment, where there may be fewer options for moving things around, at least try to position yourself so that you're not sleeping right next to a radiator. But if you must sleep beside it, try the classic apartment-dweller's remedy and put a bowl of water on top of the unit—preferably near some houseplants.

Outdoors

We're accustomed to thinking that the fresh air of the out-of-doors is good for us, and of course in many ways, it is. But did you ever go from a warm house into a cold winter morning only to find that your eyes tear? It's not that you're sad to be leaving the warmth of your home to go to work, although you may be; rather, it's that temperature and wind create a condition of dryness that stimulates the tear reflex. In the dry, scratched-up eyes of dry eye patients, that normal reaction is even more intense. What's more, dry eyes are more photo-sensitive, so bright sunlight will stimulate even graver symptoms of dry eye discomfort.

But of course, dry eye or not, you're not going to live your life in a dark, climate-controlled room with your eyes closed—even though that's an ideal condition for dry eye sufferers. Still, where and how you live and travel can have an impact on your dry eye condition.

Many of my patients here in New York City tell me that on their vacations in Florida or on a Caribbean island, their eyes felt wonderful—at least, until they went back into their air-conditioned hotel. On the beach, in the town, or walking through the rain forest, however, their dry eye symptoms seemed simply to disappear. By contrast, patients who vacation in Las Vegas or tour the desert national parks of the Southwest tell me their eyes felt miserable during their trips, despite all the wonderful sights they saw. It figures. Tropical humidity is like a warm mist for dry eyes, while desert dryness only exacerbates the condition and the symptoms.

The most important thing you can do for your eyes when you're outdoors, wherever you are and whether you have dry eye or not, is to wear sunglasses. The bigger the glasses are—the Jackie O or Bono style rather than the John Lennon granny-glasses style—and the more snug they are to the skin, the more protective they will be. They'll keep out dust, debris, allergens, and currents of dry air. Whether they're prescription, non-prescription, tinted, transitional, or clear, I can't recommend glasses highly enough.

Travel

Planes, trains, and cars are probably the worst places for any dry eye sufferer. All are closed environments in which a flow of air circulates in only a limited way. What's different about these three modes of transportation is the way dry eye sufferers can mitigate the adverse effects of the environment.

You're tooling down the Interstate. It's February, the outside temperature is two degrees Fahrenheit, and you have turned the car heater on full blast. Although the speed limit is 65, and you've set the cruise control to 70, people are passing you left, right, and center—literally. Your brain is on high alert, and you are watching the road and the other cars as hard as you can. You've got a seven-hour drive ahead of you.

Obviously, when you're behind the wheel of a car, you can't take a 10-second closed-eye break. So what can you do to alleviate the dry eye symptoms that are sure to come, given the environment you're in?

A truck driver who's a patient of mine says that when the air conditioning dries his eyes out too much, he actually slaps his face repeatedly. A less drastic move would be to direct the flow of air from the heater or air conditioner to your feet rather than at your face. You can wear sunglasses to protect your eyes from the flow of air—whether it's air from the heater/air conditioner unit or air from an open window. Even better, you can wear some version of what used to be called "motorcycle glasses." These are protective wraparound glasses—the more they wrap around, the more protective they are—and many styles offer a seal so that no air can get in, creating a kind of moisture chamber around the eyes; they are, literally, moisture chamber glasses.

And of course, you could pull off the highway, have a coffee break, stretch, and rest your eyes for a few minutes. On a long trip especially, that's a useful idea. At least make it a point to give your eyes a break every time you need to fill the tank with gas; as you stand there holding the pump, close your eyes, move them around under your closed eyelids, and let them renew their moisture.

On planes and trains, of course, you cannot pull over for a break. But unless you're the pilot or engineer, you can simply close your eyes if you're traveling the skies or rails.

A train is a slightly less closed environment than a plane; after all, trains do make stops, and doors open to let people on and off, so the air gets an occasional refreshing infusion. On the other hand, trains offer those big windows to look through. Passengers tend to stare through the glass, and they often have to concentrate hard to "catch" the scenery as it flies by. That's why dry eye sufferers should avoid looking out the window; at least, they should limit their scenery-staring and take breaks from it. The same goes for that other great railroad pastime, reading. When you read, you blink less, and since you're already in a closed environment, where you really need to blink more, take breaks from your reading as well.

Airplanes are perhaps the most unhealthy of environments for dry eye patients—in fact, for anyone. You're captive in a closed environment in which the air is constantly recycled. Hundreds of people may be passing along their various allergens through this recycled air. And it is a low-humidity environment. Above all, you can't escape—can't pull over, as in an automobile, or lean out the door between railroad cars as on a train.

Again, one thing you can do is close your eyes. You can also try to adjust the current of air from those overhead jets—yours or your neighbor's—to make sure it isn't hitting you right in the eyes. You can lubricate your eyes with cold artificial tears. And you can take breaks from reading or movie-watching.

Wearing tranquileyes is also a good bet; by sealing the area around the eyes, it approximates complete closure, and its moisture-chamber mechanism keeps the eyes humid in any event. Though they may make you look a little odd during your flight, you'll look and feel bright-eyed and rested when you arrive at your destination.

Playing Sports

Many of the "hippest" new sunglasses were originally designed for athletes—whether professionals or weekend warriors. Sports, after all, often require concentrated staring. In any game with a ball—from golf to baseball to basketball or football—the cardinal rule is to "keep your eye on the ball." Athletes often do so with ferocious intensity. Think of the golfer setting up his shot, then watching it after take-off. He is so focused on what he's doing that he is almost certainly not blinking. And he is doing all this not-blinking out in the open air, where a breeze may be carrying dust or allergens and is certainly drying out the eye's moisture.

Or consider the cyclist, whether competing in a race or just out for a day's ride. Whether she's going with or against the wind, the motion of cycling creates a current of wind blowing into the eyes, carrying with it whatever it picks up.

Is it any wonder that athletes like David Duval and Lance Armstrong wear those extra-snug wraparound glasses that keep out air and debris—and keep in moisture? And is it any wonder that week-end cyclists and golfers, not to mention baseball and football and tennis and basketball players, joggers and hikers, and just plain folks have copied those athletes' style for themselves?

It's easy to see how these glasses block the wind and seal out the dust and particles the wind may be carrying. But how do they seal in moisture? Here's how: The body radiates heat—always—but especially when you are exerting effort, as in playing sports. The heat generates moisture, and the protective sunglasses act as a shield; the radiated moist heat simply bounces off the shield and stays inside its protective bubble, keeping the protected area slightly more moist. In fact, some manufacturers of these wraparound sports glasses have introduced minuscule vents into the seal around the eyes so that the glasses don't fog up too much from the moisture within.

Protective glasses are particularly important because playing a sport or doing any physical exercise is actually good for dry eye sufferers. Of course, you don't need an eye doctor to tell you that exercise is good for you. But for dry eye sufferers, there's a particular benefit. If you're a dry eye sufferer who has ever worked out in an indoor gym, you know you never felt the discomforts of dry eye while you were exercising—unless, of course, your eyes were bothered by salty sweat dripping down from your forehead. Maybe the freedom from dry eye discomfort was because everything was flowing while you were speedwalking on the treadmill or lifting weights or pedaling hard on the stationary bike.

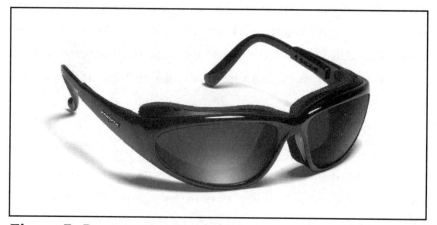

Figure 7: *Panoptx wraparound glasses*

Actually, there's a deeper reason for your eye comfort; it's the same reason all doctors tell their patients to do some form of workout regularly: exercise strengthens the immune system. Specifically, exercise strengthens the immune system's ability to fight off infection and reduce inflammation, and since inflammation is the likely cause of dry eye, people who suffer from dry eye have an extra reason to be diligent about exercising. In fact, eye have an extra reason to be diligent about exercising. In fact, the more you exercise, and the more regularly you exercise, the more you may reduce your dry eye discomfort.

Just keep in mind that staying hydrated is essential, whether your workout is in a gym or in the park. And when you do exercise in the great outdoors, wear protective glasses to shield your eyes and keep them as moist as possible.

7

YOUR LIFESTYLE AND NUTRITION

It's pretty hard these days not to know what's good for us in terms of lifestyle and nutrition. We're bombarded by headlines on an almost daily basis about the latest medical findings. And we're urged by our doctors and by our culture to stay fit, to refrain from smoking, to eat fresh rather than processed foods.

In general, what's good for overall health is good for dry eye sufferers as well: eat a healthy diet, get plenty of sleep, exercise regularly, do not smoke, take alcohol and caffeine in moderation if at all, and so on.

It's also the case for most of us, however, that we cannot totally alter our lives to meet the needs of a particular health condition. The ideal prescription for a dry eye sufferer might well be to move to a tropical jungle, stop working at the computer, quit smoking, eat fresh foods only, and live with-out stress—but it's unlikely that my patients in New York City could do all that at the drop of a hat.

Nevertheless, there are some recommendations about lifestyle behavior and nutrition that apply specifically to those of you suffering from dry eye. Many of these recommendations are about fighting inflammation, so it's important to understand what inflammation is, and why it should be fought.

Inflammation

Inflammation is one of those good news–bad news stories. The good news is that it is a normal process in which the body's white blood cells and chemicals respond to protect us against injury, infection, and such foreign intruders as bacteria and viruses. When you get a bruise, and it swells and turns red, that's evidence that all your systems are hard at work defending your body and repairing the damaged tissue.

The bad news about inflammation, however, is that it can continue beyond its normal limits or become activated to no purpose. Such inflammation is indeed unwelcome, as this normally "protective" process, with nothing to protect, actually does damage—and the response becomes worse than the stimulus that prompted it. Inflammation is now understood to be age-related as well, and it has been fingered as playing a role in a number of diseases and age-related conditions. It is also now generally agreed that it is the ultimate cause of dry eye disorder.

We are not sure precisely how all this works, but it seems clear that inflammation may be fueled by T-cells in our immune systems. In the lacrimal glands, this T-cell–inspired inflammation clogs up the tear film glands and thus blocks the secretion of tear film. Again, we do not know exactly how inflammation causes this cascade of clogging and blocking, but whatever the precise chain of events, the result is the death of cells on the eye surface and reduced quality and function in the tear film—in other words, dry eye disorders.

As for how the eye inflammation happens in the first place— how and why those T-cells get activated—again, we're not exactly sure, but any kind of immune response by the body could conceivably trigger it. That means that if you have rheumatoid arthritis or a thyroid condition or a bad cold, or if you had mononucleosis as a teenager, or if you have any sort of chronic condition—like an allergy—your eyes may be a pathway for inflammation.

Whatever the cause of the inflammation, for dry eye sufferers, there is a pretty simple bottom line: avoid what promotes inflammation, and seek out what fights inflammation. That's true in both lifestyle behaviors and nutrition.

Lifestyle Dos and Don'ts

But inflammation is not the only thing you want to fight. As you well know by now, many things can exacerbate the discomfort of dryness—and should be avoided—while there are other factors that can either soothe the dryness or advance a condition of moisture that can prevent it. So there are things you can do on a day-to-day basis that can alleviate your symptoms and help you feel and look better.

Let's start with lifestyle.

DO CATCH SOME ZZZZZS

I cannot emphasize enough how important sleep is to mitigating the discomforts of dry eye. A deep sleep of at least eight hours bathes the eye, replenishes the tear film, and soothes the ocular surface. Anything less than a long, deep sleep cheats you of those benefits and can lead to dry spots, irritation, and increased inflammation.

Napping doesn't produce quite the same benefits. It doesn't afford that long lubrication that is so refreshing and so salutary. And sometimes, napping during the day can mean less sleep at night. On the other hand, there is nothing harmful about a nap. It can renew the body, and it bathes the eyes to a certain extent. But it is nighttime sleep that really makes the difference in refreshing the ocular surface, so sleep as long and as soundly as you can.

DO EXERCISE

Regular exercise unquestionably does all sorts of good things for us—keeps us trim and limber, heightens our mood, lets the body release toxins and impurities through sweat. But as we noted in Chapter 6, the main medical benefit is perhaps the power of exercise to decrease inflammation, which it does through the release of endorphins. For that very reason, exercise contributes to the health of the ocular surface, so regular exercise—at least 20 minutes of exercise that increases your heart rate five times a week—is highly recommended for dry eye sufferers.

Do Take Showers

A hot bath can be a relaxing indulgence, but the steam tends to rise away from you, and the temperature of the water goes down by degrees as you lie there. Much better is to be upright in a shower, with steam coming at you constantly and with the temperature remaining consistently hot. Moreover, whether you intend it or not, water from the shower head or bouncing off your body splatters into your eyes and literally cleans them out. All in all, showering is as good a wash for your eyes as for your body—as well as being refreshing.

Do Drink Water

Of course, just about the best way to gain moisture is to drink it—namely in the form of from six to eight glasses of water a day. That's water—plain and simple—not sodas or sugary juices or artificially flavored drinks. Water is needed by all the body organs—by the skin, the kidneys, the liver, the heart, and the eyes as well—and it washes away the toxins and other impurities even as it helps the body perform.

Do Keep Up with Friends and Family

There is increasing evidence that social interaction—reaching out and engaging with others—is as good for us as exercise or a good night's sleep or eating nutritional foods. It lowers stress levels, takes your mind off your dry eye discomfort, and brightens your mood. It is also a fact that the smile you wear when you're with friends and feeling good can actually reduce the exposure of the ocular surface. Look in a mirror sometime when you're smiling, and you'll see the truth of this: your face scrunches up in a near-squint, and your eye closes just a bit. And the muscular function of smiling may actually release some oils onto the ocular surface as well.

DON'T GET STRESSED

Telling people to avoid stress is a little like telling them to get rich: it's a desirable outcome, but just exactly how do you go about making it happen? Of course, the bookstores and libraries are filled with books on how to reduce or manage your stress, and your own doctor can give you the best and most personal advice on the subject. The problem is that stress can affect so many of the other factors that have a direct impact on dry eye: sleep, your blink rate, even what you eat. By the same token, several of the recommendations for reducing the discomfort of dry eye—exercise, eat right, get plenty of sleep— are stress-reducers as well.

To be sure, no life is stress-free. Nor should it be. After all, stress is an atavistic response to danger, and in many ways and at many times, it can be downright good for you. But the kinds of stresses and strains that manifest themselves in tight muscles, headaches, high blood pressure, change of appetite, even gastro-intestinal problems, are the same kinds of stresses and strains that are also quite likely decreasing your blink rate, or keeping you from sleeping, or sending you to the fast-food place for dinner because you're sure you don't have time to cook a healthy meal. And all of that—decreased blinking, lack of sleep, and junk food-will lead to precisely the kind of inflammation that can exacerbate a range of ailments, including your dry eye disorder.

There are many different kinds of stress, and there are many ways to manage it. Find the ways that work for you, and learn as best you can to keep stress at a minimum. Your eyes, as well as the rest of you, will benefit when you do.

DON'T WORK YOUR EYES TOO LONG

Perhaps the most important thing to avoid if you suffer from dry eye is a long stretch of consecutive visual tasking. Whether it's working at the computer or watching television or reading, break up the time you spend doing it. Close your eyes for 10 seconds—even for 30. Get up and walk around. Hit the pause button on your DVD player and do something else for a while. It's the nonstop aspect of the visual activity that you want to guard against, not the activity itself; that consecutive streak of infrequent or no blinking means your eyes have no time to recover from being dried out. So don't give up the visual task, just interrupt the time you spend doing it.

This is particularly important at home in the evening after what may have been a tiring day at work. After an eight-hour stretch in front of the computer at the office, one of the worst things you can do for your eyes is to come home and spend two hours in front of the TV, or working at the home computer, or doing heavy reading. Instead, after a tiring day, call it quits on the staring and visual tasking; spend the time visiting with your spouse, kids, friends and neighbors, or take a walk, or consider listening to your favorite music CD in a dimly lit room. Unless you're the last living American with no way to record television programs, you probably won't miss anything you can't watch another night—and the email will still be there in the morning, too.

The reason for this recommendation is simple: if you start off with eyes already dried and irritated from the hard day at work, and you then do something that can make it worse—watching TV, reading, working at the computer—the condition will only become more severe, and the recovery will be tougher and take longer. So balance a day of heavy visual tasking with an evening of light visual tasking, if any.

DON'T SMOKE OR DRINK ALCOHOL OR CAFFEINE

Smoke, alcohol, and caffeine all dehydrate the body, including the eyes. Smoking also acts as an irritant to the eyes. Granted, all three of these activities can be habit-forming, so if you are "hooked," at least be aware of what they are doing to your dry eye disorder so you might try to reduce the frequency of your behaviors. But of course, eliminate all three if you can.

Nutrition

In 2005, Harvard's Brigham and Women's Hospital and Schepens Eye Research Institute in Boston released the findings of a study on the relationship of food to dry eye disorder. More than 32,000 women participated in the study, which found that the women who ate tuna more than five times per week had 68 percent less chance of developing dry eye than those who did not. The key ingredient that made the difference is omega-3 fatty acid, which is found not just in tuna but in other dark, coldwater fish.

OMEGA-3 AND OMEGA-6 FATTY ACIDS

Omega-3 is what is known as an essential fatty acid; that is, it cannot be produced by the body, which nevertheless requires it for the health of cells, so it must therefore be eaten in the diet. Once consumed, omega-3s block the pathways to inflammation, generate anti-inflammation agents, and promote tear secretion, so their importance for mitigating dry eye disorder is profound and unparalleled.

In fact, as the Harvard study showed, it wasn't just that omega-3s lowered the chances of getting dry eye; they also mitigated the symptoms if you already had the disorder. The study found that women with the highest levels of omega-3 in their diet had 20 percent fewer dry eye symptoms than those who had the least amount of omega-3 in their diet. Lower levels of omega-3, on the other hand, did not improve dry eye symptoms.

The study also looked at another category of essential fatty acids, the omega-6s. Omega-6 fats are found in great abundance in the American diet because they are key ingredients in ice cream sundaes, pizza, cheeseburgers, Twinkies, and other junk food—all staples, it would seem, of our national eating.

What the Harvard study concluded is that a higher dietary ratio of omega-6 fatty acid to omega-3 fatty acid raised the chance of getting dry eye, while a lower ratio of omega-6s to omega-3s lowered the likelihood. In fact, a dietary ratio of omega-6 to omega-3 greater than 15 to 1 meant a 2.5-fold increased risk of dry eye syndrome in women, according to the study. That's key, because the American diet typically has just about that ratio of omega-6 to omega-3 fats—about 15 to 1. That tells us that we need to shift that ratio significantly if we are to beat dry eye.

Does this mean that we should all eat tuna, known to be high in omega-3s, five times a week? Unfortunately, there's a serious problem with that idea—namely, the high levels of mercury, a potential health risk, in tuna, as well as in mackerel, sardines, herring, and other fish. Yes, the risk is lower if the fish are wild and not farm-raised, and it is lower still from Pacific and Alaskan fish than from Atlantic catches. Still, the recommendation from our Food & Drug Administration, watchdog of food safety, is to limit our intake of fish like farmed salmon or tuna—even canned tuna—to just once a week.

A better idea may be to take fish oil supplements. These supply the omega-3 fatty acids, sometimes in combination with other ingredients, without the risk of mercury. But it's important to get your supplements from a reputable supplier, one that obtains its oils from wild fish and that maintains a purification or filtration system. My own brand of supplement, known as Dry-Vites, is a combination of wild salmon oil and flaxseed oil, the latter being another excellent source of omega-3 fatty acids, and the production process is carefully and rigorously supervised for safety and purity. TheraTears and Biosyntrx also make fish oil products, as do other reputable manufacturers, so it is not difficult to find supplements of good quality and reliability.

In addition to certain fish, a number of foods are rich in omega-3s, including soybean and soybean oil, wheat germ, walnuts, flaxseed, and canola oil-to name a few.

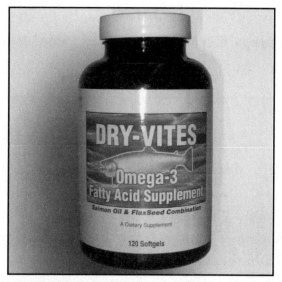

Figure 8: *Dry-Vites, an excellent source of omega-3 fatty acids*

An Anti-Inflammation Diet

While omega-3 fatty acids are the only substances known specifically to have a direct impact on the dry eye disorder, a diet that is rich in anti-inflammation foods and that avoids foods that promote inflammation will help alleviate dry eye symptoms. Although anti-inflammation diets—also called anti-aging diets—have become something of a recent fad, they represent a healthy way of eating that is hardly new.

The following foods cause inflammation:

- White foods, like dairy, sugar, and refined grains (but not eggs)
- High-carbohydrate foods
- Low-protein foods
- Foods rich in omega-6 fatty acids, like safflower, sunflower, and corn oils, mayonnaise, creamy salad dressings, meat, and peanuts

- And worst of all, trans fats—vegetable shortenings and hard margarines and just about all processed foods, which rely on hydrogenated oils to extend their shelf life

---

Throw It Out!

It's a good idea to throw out anything in your pantry or fridge that contains hydrogenated or partially hydrogenated oils. These are the trans fats, and even if you think the foods they are in taste good, you'll lose your appetite for them when you realize they do nothing but harm to your health in general and to the health of your eyes in particular. We need fats in our diet, but the trans fats have no redeeming qualities whatsoever. Stick to foods that offer omega-3 fatty acids—and throw your trans fat foods out of your kitchen and out of your life.

By contrast, the foods that fight inflammation are leafy green and brightly pigmented vegetables as well as fruits of every variety—and of course, fish.

Bottom line: avoid the foods in the bulleted list as much as you can. Have fish once a week, and eat all you can of colorful fruits and vegetables. You'll be helping your overall health, your longevity, and of course your eyes when you do.

VITAMINS FOR DRY EYE?

A number of vitamin products now on the supermarket and drugstore shelves claim to be good for eye health. One formula,

---

The Health Food Way

Specialized health foods may reduce the risk of dry eye and alleviate its symptoms even more. For one thing, unprocessed foods—the core promise of the organic food industry—is far better for you than processed food. Organic product lines eschew growth hormones and pesticides, which promote inflammation. And your local health food store is more likely to stock olive oil that is truly cold-pressed and monounsaturated fats from fruits, avocados, canola, almonds, apricots, thus extending your range of choices. In addition, you can often find such items as eggs enriched with omega-3 fatty acids—a powerhouse of inflammation fighters.

---

targeted at people suffering from age-related macular degeneration, a major cause of blindness, combines vitamins A, C, and E, plus copper and zinc. The formula has been shown to achieve a 25 percent reduction in the progression of the disease in intermediate or advanced cases. That is very hopeful news, but it has nothing to do with dry eye. Certainly, if you have been diagnosed with macular degeneration, or if members of your family have had the disease, you should consult with your doctor about taking this vitamin formula. But no studies have as yet shown that it works for dry eye, and so far, it has had no effect on dry eye symptoms in any of my patients.

Other supplements promise relief from dry eye specifically through high doses of vitamin E. Vitamin E is both a much used

---

Vitamin A

In many third-world countries, a deficiency of vitamin A has been identified as a leading cause of dry eye. That is not a problem in the American diet, where vitamin A is routinely ingested via such foods as carrots, liver, sweet potatoes, eggs, milk, cantaloupe, and spinach.

---

and hotly debated supplement, but it is important to know what kind of vitamin E you're taking—and how much. There are actually different types of vitamin E, and while the alpha-tocopherol type is good for some things—it fights the aging process and may protect against some cancers—it has no effect on dry eye; for that, you want the gamma-tocopherol type.

In addition, too much vitamin E, even in cases where it may have a beneficial effect, can actually be toxic. A recent study, for example, found that people who took 400 International Units of E per day—most multivitamins contain 40 IU—were five percent more likely to die than those taking placebos. So be wary of any supplement that claims to offer a large amount of vitamin E, or of any kind of supplement. A large amount may be way too much. Stick to what you get in foods like nuts, wheat germ, soybean and canola oil, shrimp, sweet potatoes, broccoli, spinach, garbanzo beans, mangoes, eggs, sunflower seeds, avocados, tomatoes, and asparagus—and supplement that, if at all, with a multivitamin.

It's not easy to make changes in lifestyle behaviors. It's often downright hard to change your diet or a habitual way of eating. But making any of the changes recommended in this chapter can help your dry eye—possibly significantly. And certainly, doing everything recommended here will make a difference you'll feel and see.

8

YOUR HOME EYE SPA

Home can and should be the epicenter of restoring eye health, for it's here that you spend most of your time (especially sleep time), and it's here that you should feel most comfortable.

It's at home, too, in the privacy of your bathroom or bedroom, that you can learn how to do the simple cleansing treatment I call the Home Eye Spa. The Home Eye Spa is really the front line of the battle against dry eye discomfort, as you gently clean your eyes and unclog the glands that literally oil the tear film. You'll find detailed instructions for the Home Eye Spa, with illustrations, later in the chapter. First, however, refer back to what you learned about the environment in Chapter 6 and ensure that your home itself is not exacerbating your dry eye condition.

The Home Eye Spa

With your home environment adjusted as well as possible to bolster your eye comfort, not detract from it, you'll be well positioned to get the most out of the Home Eye Spa procedure. Originally, I designed the procedure for patients suffering from blepharitis, meibomian gland dysfunction, and rosacea, but it works for anyone who suffers from dry eye, whether it's caused by these or any other conditions. What's more, it's an extremely effective preventive for all these disorders, and it's beneficial for the health of your eyes in general. Here's what it's about:

Remember the meibomian glands you were introduced to back in Chapter 1? There are some 50 of them along the margins of both the top and bottom eyelids. With every blink of your eye, these glands pump oily, lipid-like secretions onto the top of your tear film. This oil coats the tear film, serving as its top protective layer and preventing it from evaporating.

Until and unless the meibomian glands get clogged up. When that happens, the tear film of course evaporates more rapidly, and the result is dryness, burning, irritation—all the disorders of tear-film dysfunction.

We call the condition blepharitis, which simply means eyelid inflammation. Blepharitis is a common cause of dry eye, although it is possible to have dry eye without blepharitis—and blepharitis treatments may not be necessary in that case. It manifests itself in all the kinds of symptoms we've recorded in this book, symptoms that are very familiar to just about everyone over the age of 40: redness, difficulty wearing contact lenses, dryness or tearing, intermittently blurry vision, bags under the eyes, crusty eyes in the morning. The very fact that these are pretty ordinary irritations means that people tend not to pay too much attention to them at first, with the unhappy result that the condition continues to worsen, becoming harder and harder to treat.

In addition, as you know, skin conditions like rosacea, as well as dandruff, psoriasis, eczema, and so forth, can exacerbate the condition and irritate the blepharitis even further. Often, patients will focus on the skin condition and forget about the eye disorder—which again just lets the condition worsen over time. One thing patients with skin conditions should certainly be aware of is to avoid alcohol-based or heavily fragrant skin products. Look for hypo-allergenic products instead.

There is no cure for blepharitis, but it can be easily managed by the basic Home Eye Spa treatment. In fact, I recommend the basic treatment for everyone 25 and older, because treating the skin conditions can mitigate the worst effects of dry eye later in life. There's nothing sadder than to see a 70-year-old patient who has been suffering the symptoms of blepharitis for decades without knowing it. It is much harder to treat this person—and it will take much longer for him to feel relief—than if he had been following the basic Home Eye Spa treatment routinely. Bottom line? Try to make the treatment as regular a part of your personal care regimen as flossing your teeth, or giving yourself an exfoliating facial, or doing your nails—three times a week if you can.

What You'll Need

The treatment focuses on cleaning the eyelids using heat, massage, and a gentle cleansing procedure. I use a heat pad, called the Eye Spa Pad, that conforms to the shape of the eye; pop it in a microwave for 30 seconds, and it will stay hot for five minutes—sufficient time to loosen the glands, step one in the cleansing process. The pad also has a soft cotton exterior, which is important since you will be placing it on your face, and the exterior is washable, which is important because you will sweat under the heat, and the pad can become dirty after a number of uses. The pad can also be cooled—just put it in the refrigerator—so that you can use it to soothe red, inflamed, irritated eyes. It's thus a multi-use piece of gear—one that you can re-use time and again.

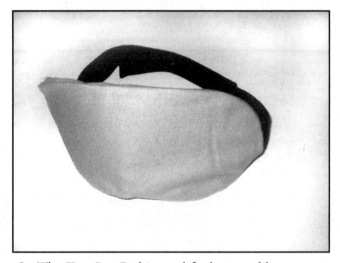

Figure 9: *The Eye Spa Pad is good for hot or cold treatments*

But you don't need to use my heat pad. Warm compresses will also work, and a facecloth will do in a pinch, although warmth in either of those lasts for only seconds.

In addition to the compress or heat pad, you will need cotton swabs—the sterilized kind are best—and at least two vials of preservative-free eye drops that you have stashed in a corner of your refrigerator to cool.

Two cautions: First, gentleness is extremely important in doing the basic Home Eye Spa treatment. Too often, doctors will recommend that patients perform an eyelid "scrub." But "scrub" is not a good word here; it sounds rough, even abrasive, and any such action can further irritate the eye and will stretch and wrinkle the skin. So be gentle every step of the way. And of course remember never to touch the eyeball itself.

Second, it's very important to do this procedure right. I know that many doctors just hand patients a photocopied list of instructions for their eyelid "scrub" and tell them to "go home and try it." Most end up using a lid scrub from Ocusoft, or they might turn to a fantastic new product from TheraTears called Steri-Lids. While these products are superficial cleansers, they can help if used correctly. But to really do the job right, a little pressure—and a little focus—are definitely needed.

In fact, trying the procedure without seeing it isn't very effective, which is why my instructions below are accompanied by illustrations. I urge you to follow the instructions to the letter; doing the treatment incorrectly is as bad as not doing anything. It may take a number of tries to get it right, but it is worth the effort to do so, for the results will be highly beneficial—not just in terms of comfort, but in treating your dry eye disorder.

Ready? Let's learn the basic Home Eye Spa treatment.

Treatment Basics

Remember when you were a teenager worried about pimples? You took time every now and again to "treat" them. Remember how? First, you washed your face with water as hot as you could stand to soften up the pimple and loosen the pus inside. Then you popped and squeezed. Then you wiped away the pus and rinsed your face again. The same principle is at work in unclogging the meibomian glands.

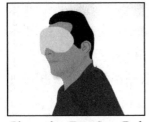

Place the Eye Spa Pad over your closed eyes.

Step 1. Heat first. The point is to loosen the gunk that may be plugged up in the meibomian glands and to open the clogged ducts. Sometimes, in fact, the heat alone can unclog the glands and restore function. Heat up the Eye Spa Pad (or a moistened towel), check with your fingers that it's not too hot, lie down on your bed or on a sofa, apply the pad to your eyes, and just relax for three minutes. While you're relaxing, the heat from the pad is working to open the ducts of the meibomian glands and loosen the contents, and to open the pores of your skin and loosen any debris there.

Step 2. Next comes massage. Gently pull your eyelid slightly to the side. Then take a cotton swab dipped in hot water, and, starting at the nose-end of your eye, gently push at the lower eyelid margin just below the eyelash. Basically, you're pressing the eyelid ever so delicately against the eyeball, and this serves to push

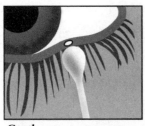

Gently massage your eyelid with a cotton swab.

the contents of the meibomian glands up and out of the ducts. Do this very softly all along the bottom eyelid margin. Then, again starting at the nose, do the same thing on the top eyelid margin, pressing right above the eyelash line to express the contents of the upper eyelid glands down and out. This is all very gentle and very quick; it shouldn't take more than 10 seconds or so.

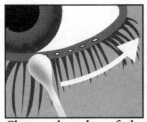

Cleanse the edge of the eyelid margin gently with a cotton swab.

Step 3. Now we cleanse the eyelid. Simply take the cotton swab and with one stroke, gently wipe the eyelid below the eyelash line for the upper eyelid, above it for the lower eyelid. You're simply wiping away the gunk you've squeezed out of the eyelid margins, just as you once scrubbed off the pus from a popped pimple. Do NOT wipe *inside* your eyelid!

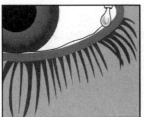

Place several cold preservative-free eye drops in each eye.

Step 4. For the final clean-up, take those preservative-free or disappearing-preservative eye drops out of the refrigerator and apply about five drops per eye—that's typically one vial of the preservative-free drops. You want to rinse out of your eye everything you may have stirred up with the heat and/or the massage; indeed, it's important to wash all that residual debris out of there. And it will also feel nice and soothing.

All in all, the basic eye spa home treatment should take no more than five minutes or so. I recommend that when you first begin the treatment, you do it on a daily basis. This kind of regular practice will help you get good at it and will begin to plant the habit. Once you've got it down pat, keep it up at least three times a week.

Actually, even if you don't achieve total mastery, the heat pad alone can make an enormous difference in just loosening the glands and opening the passageways out of your eyelids. So doing just Step 1 of the Home Eye Spa treatment is better than doing nothing for both preventive and therapeutic purposes.

And while you will not notice instant relief, the treatment does bring improvement in due course. Yes, it takes time to reverse the accumulated ill effects of the condition, but it does happen—if you do the treatment on a steadily consistent basis. How long until you notice a change? Janet, a 65-year-old patient of mine who was greatly bothered by her red, puffy eyelid margins and the loss of her eyelashes, applied herself to learn and perform the basic Home Eye Spa treatment assiduously. Within six months, the redness and puffiness were gone, and she stopped losing lashes; in fact, her eyelashes looked thicker than ever. For Janet, a woman of great determination who had risen through the corporate ranks during a successful career in financial services, this was an incentive to continue the basic eye spa home treatment religiously. And while her improved appearance may be what's making her happiest, as her physician, I am thrilled by the improvement in her tear film function.

But if you simply cannot follow any sort of regimen—or if you just balk at the idea—here's the lazy person's version of the Home Eye Spa treatment:

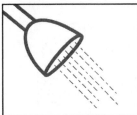

Step 1. Either do Step 1 of the treatment, placing the heat pad on your eyes for three minutes of delicious relaxation, or take a long, hot shower.

Take a hot shower.

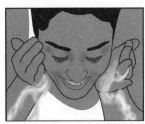

Step 2. Once the heat has loosened the contents of the meibomian glands, use just the ball of your finger to gently massage the edges of your eyelids, as shown.

Apply gentle pressure to the edges of your eyelids with your fingers.

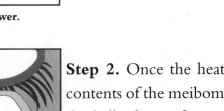

Step 3. Rinse your face thoroughly with cold water; this constricts the blood vessels and makes your eyes and face look better. If you're in the shower, try letting the flow of the water bounce off your hand into your eyes. This is a good rinse, and by having it bounce off the hand, you lessen the force of the water.

Gently rinse your eyes with cool water.

Cool Tips

Store some gel compresses, like my Soothers, in the refrigerator. Then, whenever your eyes feel irritated, sore, or tired, pull out a pair, apply, and chill out. The

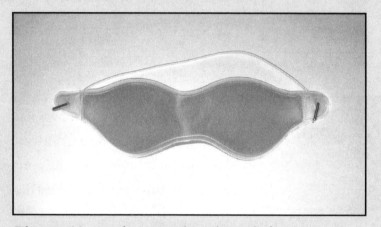

Figure 10: *Soothers provide cooling relief*

simple result is constriction of the blood vessels, but the sensation is remarkably soothing.

But there's more to it than that. Want to save yourself the cost of those expensive creams and salves you buy to try to deflate the bags under your eyes—not to mention the last-resort choice of cosmetic surgery to get rid of them? Just make it a habit to apply cold Soothers or other gel packs on those dark bags under the eyes. This will reduce the inflammation that is so irritating—and that you tend to exacerbate by rubbing—and will in time reduce the bags themselves. You'll feel good doing something about your appearance, and you'll feel great when you see the bags shrink to nothing.

PART THREE

BEYOND THE HOME EYE SPA

In addition to your Home Eye Spa treatments, you and your eye doctor may well have determined that your dry eye requires medical therapy. In that case, it's important to remember that the body is a system and that therapeutic action on one part of the system can easily affect any other part of the system. Chapter 9 tells how any treatments you might be taking—from an over-the-counter cold remedy to a physician-prescribed heart medicine—may affect or be affected by a course of treatment for your dry eye.

As an example of how all things in the body are interconnected, current research is showing an undeniable link between hormones and dry eye, and this presages lots of new possibilities for treatment. Chapter 10 alerts you to hormone-based eye drops now in the pipeline that may make an important difference to dry eye sufferers in the not-too-distant future.

But beyond drugs and drops, there are other treatment solutions for dry eye as well. In Chapter 11, you'll learn about the use of punctal plugs, a key remedy for dry eye, and other means of keeping the tearsin without drugs. Finally, Chapter 11 describes the various options available should surgery become necessary.

9

MEDICINES THAT HELP, MEDICINES THAT HARM

One of the toughest things about my practice is to see people who have suffered dry eye for years without any viable solution. They have tried one thing and another, spent a fortune, and had no lasting success.

The failure shows. The eyes of these people can look bleary at best, red and, irritated at worst, while the skin around their eyes is wrinkled, swollen, and raw. There's pain involved as well, as they deal day after day with a discomfort that has them rubbing their eyes, squinting, and looking as downcast as they feel.

The eye doctors who have tried to help these patients have had to do so with one hand tied behind their backs, for medical research has historically focused its resources on other, more "dramatic" eye issues over the years. Increasingly, however, tear film disorders have become the subject of scientific scrutiny and experiment, with the result, at long last, that pharmaceutical companies have begun to develop treatment products specific to dry eye and its related problems.

In fact, there is a newly emerging set of treatments, both topical and oral, that offer a range of options eye doctors can prescribe to address dry eye conditions and disorders. This is very good news indeed for dry eye sufferers, so long as they keep in mind that there is no single "cure" that fits every condition or disorder. Still, the chances are good that one of the options now available can be prescribed to treat your dry eye disorder.

At the same time, before I prescribe any treatment for my patients, I need to know what other medications, if any, they may be taking—not just to relieve their dry eye but for any health condition whatsoever. This is, or should be, standard operating procedure for any responsible physician. There are so many potential interactions among different pills, drops, liquids, and even salves, whatever their purpose, that it simply makes no sense to prescribe a treatment without having the total picture in hand first. Without such a complete profile on a patient's medications, a doctor might order up a treatment that interacts with another in such a way as to cause a dangerous side effect—or one treatment may simply cancel out the benefits of another.

Remember Susan from Chapter 4 with her sack of medications all interacting in toxic ways to make her eyes almost unbearably irritated? She did the right thing in bringing the whole collection with her when she came to my office for her appointment—and I recommend you follow her lead. When you visit your doctor, bring either a list of all your medications, or just bring the medications themselves.

For the fact is that dry eye can indeed be caused or exacerbated by a number of fairly common treatments that are routinely prescribed for patients or that patients may be taking on their own—everything from over-the-counter cold medicines to herbal supplements to essential medications for high blood pressure. Certainly, you can't stop taking your blood-pressure medicine because you have dry eye. Instead, it's the physician's task to create a therapy that accommodates both needs. That's why, as important as it is to know about the medicines that can help heal dry eye, it's equally important to know about those that may make it worse. This chapter informs you about both.

The New Drug That Makes Tears

The skies were overcast the day Barbara first came to my office. Nevertheless, she wore a large black picture hat with a floppy brim and huge and very dark sunglasses big enough to cover much of her face. Although not a particularly tall woman, she kept her head tilted down, as if she were looking at my desk, not at me. It gave her a dejected appearance that her stern and unsmiling manner only exaggerated. When I asked her to remove the hat, take off the sunglasses, and look up at me, I could see why she always hid or averted her eyes: they were beet-red with irritation, and the skin around them appeared broken, scratched, and flaky. Barbara looked, in short, to be in pain. She also looked 20 years older than her actual age. The hat and the sunglasses partly obscured these realities, but they couldn't end them—which was why her mood was as dark as her oversized designer shades.

More than one doctor had diagnosed Barbara's condition as allergic and had prescribed anti-allergy medicines. The diagnosis was correct; she did have allergies. What had been missed, however, was that she also had dry eye, and the allergy medicines, while treating the allergic condition, were actually exacerbating the tear film disorder and making her dry eyes even drier.

In my view, Barbara was a candidate for the new tear-making wonder drug created by Allergan, Restasis, the most prominent and potentially the most effective of the new treatments coming out of the pharmaceutical company labs. As of this writing, Restasis is the only FDA-approved eye drop that actually makes your eye make more tears, and while similar treatments are said to be in the pipeline, to date, there is nothing else like Restasis available.

The key ingredient in Restasis is cyclosporine, which it contains in only a minute amount; in fact, only 0.05 percent of a Restasis dose is cyclosporine. Yet even that tiny amount is sufficient to prevent the activation of T-cells, which is precisely what Restasis—and only Restasis—does. The result is that it is a medicine that keeps the lacrimal glands from getting clogged up, and they can therefore make tears normally.

Barbara's irritated, inflamed eyes looked to me to have precisely the kind of inflammation-induced dry eye disorder that Restasis was meant for. And in fact, its effectiveness in the case of "quieter" pictures of dry eye is limited; it simply wasn't made for these less excited-looking, if equally uncomfortable, disorders. As a result, it brings to them an overkill impact that achieves little if any relief. But for eyes like Barbara's, Restasis goes right to the cause of the discomfort and can be highly effective. And unlike steroids, the typical anti-inflammation treatment, Restasis has not been found to have any systemic medical side effects.

For patients eager to see and feel results, however, there is a kind of psychological downside to Restasis—namely, it takes a number of weeks for it to really start working. The reason is that the cyclosporine has no effect on T-cells that are already activated; it simply prevents the activation of any "future" T-cells. So it is going to take at least four weeks—even as many as six—for the effects of the already activated T-cells to peter out. Then and only then will the blocking impact of Restasis kick in.

Moreover, in the first month of using Restasis, some patients may feel symptoms that result directly from the drug itself—burning, redness, itchiness, even some vision blurring and the occasional sensation of a foreign object in the eye. Frustrated because there is no instant gratification in terms of relief, some patients may actually "fail therapy," as the term goes; that is, they simply give up on the drug before it has had its chance to do its job—a real shame, particularly because Restasis is typically covered by insurance.

That's why, in Barbara's case, I made sure to be very clear with her about what to expect in terms of impact and time. I told her not to expect anything for the first four to six weeks—except some possible symptoms of discomfort—and I alerted her to the reality that she probably wouldn't experience the peak effects of Restasis for about four months. Be patient, I counseled her; it will be worth it. Barbara agreed that the time and discomfort would indeed be worth accepting if she could get relief.

In addition to setting the stage in terms of expectations, I sought to mitigate what we might call the "annoyance factor"—the early discomforts and the need for patience—by prescribing a very diluted steroid, Lotemax, by Bausch & Lomb, which I had Barbara take for the first four weeks as she was beginning the Restasis regimen. The reason? As the classic anti-inflammatories, steroids attack another of those inflammation pathways—a different pathway from the one the cyclosporine in the Restasis works on—and thus they counter the initial discomfort the Restasis produces. But of course, steroids do carry a number of side effects, so although they can perform wonders in the short term, they must be used just that way—on a short-term basis only. The Lotemax I prescribed for Barbara—and prescribe for many patients on Restasis—would give the Restasis time to kick in while helping turbocharge the fight against the inflammation. The purpose is psychological as much as anything; the aim of the Lotemax is to get people more comfortable with Restasis so they won't fail therapy—and fail to experience the truly beneficial effects of this drug.

In addition, I advised Barbara to stop taking the allergy medicines she was ingesting orally, instead prescribing a topical salve to soothe the irritation she felt without exacerbating the disorder.

Four months later, on a brilliantly sunny autumn day, Barbara showed up at my office with no hat, no sunglasses, her head held high, and a broad smile on her face. She looked and felt 20 years younger, and you could see it in the clear, smooth skin of her face and sense it in the bounce in her step. "You've made the whites of my eyes white again," she announced happily. Her pain and discomfort were entirely gone, as were the red eyes and wrinkled skin.

Three years later, still on Restasis and topical allergy drops (both applied twice a day) and of course still practicing her Home Eye Spa treatments, Barbara is a woman who feels her life has been changed. She finds the Restasis easy to deal with and knows that it is addressing the cause of her problem in order to eliminate its effects on her comfort and her appearance. To her, that makes it a miracle drug.

More Meds for Dry Eye

As of this writing, Allergan's Restasis stands alone as the tear-making medication for dry eye sufferers, although the pharmaceutical industry has announced that a number of other prescription drops are under development and expected to be on the market by 2015, if not sooner.

But effective as it is, the tear-producer is not the only treatment for dry eye sufferers. In fact, depending on the individual's particular disorder-not to mention the other medications the person may be taking-other treatments that work in other ways can produce similarly successful results.

One of those is a very common family of antibiotics, the tetracycline family that includes doxycycline and minocycline. Certainly, many people are reluctant to use antibiotics—rightly so—because far too many types of bacteria can become resistant to these medicines. But for certain dry eye sufferers, these antibiotics work as highly effective anti-inflammatories, not as bacteria-killers.

Rick was a perfect candidate for this treatment, and it has worked perfectly for him. He's 27, a graduate student in electrical engineering, and a chronic rosacea sufferer. Like most people afflicted with rosacea, he gets a real flare-up of the disease if he's anywhere near caffeine, alcohol, or smoky rooms—things most graduate students cannot avoid. The severe acne that such flare-ups produce has affected him profoundly, giving him a hangdog look and an understandably reserved approach to people. And the ocular rosacea that is an inevitable condition of the disease had begun to affect his ability to do his work; recurrent inflammation and scarring of the cornea meant he simply couldn't see well enough to see the blackboard with ease during class lectures—a situation exacerbated further by his spending much of every day staring at a computer, and therefore not blinking nearly as much as he should.

Rick had seen a number of doctors, but none of the treatments they prescribed had worked. He was depressed, frustrated, and ashamed of the way he looked when he came to see me.

Rick's problem—and the problem for most people with rosacea or blepharitis—is that the eyelids are chronically inflamed. That means that the meibomian glands in the eyelids that produce and discharge the essential, lubricating, oily component of the tear film are not functioning normally. When the glands are inflamed, they become clogged, and the clear lubricating oil, unable to flow, becomes stagnant and milky—no kind of lubricant at all. The tetracycline family of antibiotics works as an anti-inflammatory for the eyelids, unclogging the meibomian glands so they can pump out oil normally.

I prescribed a six-week course of doxycycline for Rick, and in only three weeks, the difference was noticeable: both his ocular rosacea and his facial acne had cleared considerably, and there was a smile on his face. After three months of treatment, the results were so good that Rick was down to one pill a day—plus cleansing and regular Home Eye Spa treatments—and it was clear he could get off the antibiotics and rely solely on the Home Eye Spa soon. Above all, he felt restored and refreshed, and he was back to his normal level of 27-year-old-graduate-student activity. While Rick could conceivably have to come back for repeat treatments in the future, he is confident that he can get relief and restore his life through this kind of treatment.

True, there can be downsides to treatment with antibiotics; side effects can occur, and of course prolonged use, repeated use, or misuse can lead to antibiotic resistance. But for rosacea sufferers like Rick, or for folks who simply cannot tolerate eye drops, or for anyone with chronic eyelid inflammation, the tetracyclines work wonderfully well—and are covered by insurance carriers across the board.

Two More Possibilities

If you have an easy time as a blood donor, you might be a candidate for what is called autologous serum eye drops. Made from your own blood, which is specially collected and spun fast to separate the red cells from the serum, these drops naturally contain such ingredients as protein and growth factors that lubricate the surface of your eye and heal the tear film.

Autologous serum eye drops are a way of treating dry eye with your body's own defense system, which appeals to many patients. It means you're not really using a drug, and there are no preservatives or additives in the eye drops; it's just your autologous serum diluted with saline.

The problem with this treatment is that you have to draw your blood every couple of months or so. You'll also need to take care with your supply of eye drops, which must be kept refrigerated and need to remain sterile. Still, studies are showing some definite benefits from this treatment, and it is one of which dry eye sufferers should be aware.

There is also some evidence that two agents prescribed for dry mouth may work for dry eye as well. These are salagen, the active ingredient of which is pilocarpine, and cevimeline. Both are prescribed routinely for Sjögren's Syndrome patients, all of whom suffer from dry mouth, which the two agents treat by stimulating secretions from the salivary glands. The emerging evidence offers some indication that both may also stimulate secretion from the lacrimal glands and thus improve the tear film. While the jury is still out on the final verdict for salagen and cevimeline as dry eye healers, those who suffer from the condition should be aware of their potential.

The Unlucky Seven: Medicines That Might Make Your Dry Eye Worse

As a doctor, I'm acutely aware of the first rule of the Hippocratic Oath: Do no harm. Certainly, medical science has developed—and continues to develop-a range of products that can soothe and heal dry eye conditions. But many medicines developed to heal other diseases and disorders can actually harm dry eye sufferers. Awareness is the essential first step toward dealing with this dilemma, so it's important for patients to be aware of both the medicines that heal and the medicines that may harm you.

There are at least seven categories of medicines that can be harmful for dry eye sufferers:

- Antihistamines/decongestants
- Anti-depressants, anti-psychotics, and sleeping pills
- Diuretics
- Beta-blockers
- Oral contraceptives and hormone treatments
- Urinary bladder control medicines
- Accutane and other systemic retinoids
- Over-the-counter drops that claim they will "get the red out" or relieve irritation

Although we're not sure exactly why and how, all these categories of treatment do seem to worsen the dryness in some way. If that sounds vague, the truth is that as far as we've come in understanding and treating dry eye, there's still an awful lot about it we just don't know. We're still discovering the different pathways along which the disorder gets going and the various mechanisms by which it works. But if we're not one hundred percent sure how these categories of treatment cause or exacerbate dry eye, we do know for sure that there is a connection: these types of medication can cause or exacerbate dry eye disorders.

In fact, in addition to these seven categories of treatment, there are other categories of medicine that probably exacerbate dry eye as well—among them thyroid medicines and treatments for erectile dysfunction. And there is a whole other region of therapies—natural and herbal supplements and homeopathic remedies—that, as we have seen, are beyond the reach of government regulation and that may contain ingredients that harm your dry eye, but there's simply no way of knowing.

Of course, this doesn't mean you should give up your heart medication, or avoid your morning vitamins and supplements, or that you'd be willing to relinquish Viagra! But it's a good idea to keep in mind that a whole range of treatments may be affecting your dry eye adversely. That's why your physician needs to know exactly what treatments you use—pills, ointments, supplements, everything. I know that I use such information both in making a diagnosis and in recommending one particular dry eye treatment over another. And if I feel that your particular dry eye condition requires a therapy that is at odds with another important therapy you're receiving, that's when I'll want to consult with your internist, or cardiologist, or gynecologist. There may be an alternate dose or alternate medicine that can achieve the same endpoint without causing or contributing to your dry eye.

So be aware of what medicines you're taking and of their potential effects on your body in all cases, and for dry eye sufferers, keep a special watch on these medications:

Antihistamines/decongestants. Whether your doctor has given you a prescription or you've bought over-the-counter relief for your stuffed head and runny nose, all antihistamines and decongestants are essentially drying agents. That's how they make you feel better—they dry your runny nose and stuffed-up sinuses, and at the same time, of course, they dry out your eyes.

But while you may get some solace out of these agents when you have a cold, dry eye sufferers should stay away from them as "allergy" medications. Chances are the "allergy" is a misdiagnosis of your dry eye, so in this case, the "cure" only makes the disease worse. Remember Barbara at the beginning of this chapter? She was a classic example of someone who had both allergies and dry eye, and the allergy medicines were canceling out her dry eye treatments by actually making the dry eye worse. In her case, we were able to find an effective alternative to her allergy medicines—a topical salve—while treating the real underlying problem, her dry eye disorder.

Anti-depressants, anti-psychotics, and sleeping pills. Here's another classic case where we physicians need to consider the total-health picture and work around two conflicting therapies. These all-important medicines can indeed decrease tear production, but they are crucial to the general well-being of the patient. Ophthalmologists must therefore consider all the options available in prescribing dry eye treatment for patients who take these drugs.

Diuretics. Ditto for diuretics, which can play an important role in stabilizing blood pressure. We really don't know why, but epidemiological studies make it pretty clear that these medicines decrease tear production.

Beta-blockers. These medications, also used for high blood pressure and heart disease, also seem to stymie tear production, although again, we don't know for sure exactly how.

Oral contraceptives and hormone treatments. Some hormones can regulate fluid production to suppress inflammation, so an imbalance in hormone levels can cause some enzymes to be more active than others, and that, in turn, promotes dry eye. As we'll learn in greater detail in Chapter 9, androgens, the male hormones, seem to protect against this dryness more than do estrogens, but there's still controversy about the impact of estrogen-only hormone replacement therapy and estrogen-combination replacements. This helps explain the reality every dry eye doctor confronts—that most dry eye patients are older females in whom androgen levels are diminishing. It is also why some pharmaceutical companies are researching the possible use of androgens in dry eye treatment. See Chapter 9 for much more on this subject.

Urinary bladder control medicines. These medicines work to block the release of tears. Specifically, they act as anticholinergics, and cholinergics are neurotransmitters found throughout the body that stimulate the production and secretion of tears, saliva, even the digestive acids in the stomach. You may be taking an anticholinergic to control your bladder secretions, but of course your body doesn't know that, so the anticholinergic will also affect your tear film secretions—and exacerbate your dry eye condition.

Accutane and other systemic retinoids. If you have severe acne and are taking a systemic retinoid like Accutane, it will also affect the meibomian glands in your eyelids, harming the quality of your tear film and potentially limiting the quantity of tear film secreted as well.

Over-the-counter eye drops. As you learned in Chapter 4, too many of the over-the-counter, quick-fix eye drops that promise to lessen irritation and reduce redness can do just the opposite. They don't address the underlying problem at all, the preservatives in them can produce a rebound redness and irritation, and they can become almost addictive, thus exacerbating your dry eye regularly and ever more painfully.

If you do take these drops now and again for quick relief, be sure not to apply them right after applying other dry eye medications—Restasis, for example—as they may wash the medication right out of the eye.

If you take any of these medications and suffer from dry eye, let both your eye doctor and your other doctors know. If you don't take them and you suffer from dry eye, be forewarned.

In general, it's best to avoid them. They're not a long-term solution.

1 0

HORMONE THERAPY FOR DRY EYES

That there is a link between hormones and dry eye is now indisputable, although the precise nature of the link and the mechanism by which hormonal activity affects the eye's moisture are still not perfectly understood. The evidence of the link is so compelling, however, that pharmaceutical companies have put the development of hormone-based dry eye treatments on the fast track. In my view, this is all happening not a moment too soon, for it is clear to me that hormones will play a significant role in the treatment of dry eyes in the future.

The studies that have compiled the inescapable evidence on hormones have focused on both estrogen and androgen. As you remember from your high-school biology course, estrogen is the primary female hormone, while androgen is the basic male hormone. Both types of hormone are found in both men and women, but, at the most basic level, estrogen is present at a far greater level in women and androgen at a far higher level in men.

The Estrogen Connection

The first real hint of the connection between these hormones and dry eye came in the landmark studies of 2002 on women and HRT—the hormone replacement therapy that had long been touted as a panacea for the discomforts, distresses, and susceptibility to diseases experienced by so many women during and after menopause. Menopause, marked by the end of a woman's reproductive capability and the cessation of her menstruation, typically produces hot flashes, night sweats, difficulty sleeping, mood changes, and vaginal dryness, and the replacement of fading hormones was seen not only as a "cure" for these conditions but also as having the bonus functions of preventing heart disease, osteoporosis, various forms of cancer, even dementia.

By 2002, a huge number of women in the U.S. were taking HRT. It was estimated that some 38 percent of all post-menopausal women in the U.S. were on a daily pill regimen of a hormone replacement that combined synthetic estrogen and progesterone-progestin—while millions more were on an estrogen-only regimen. So it was a shock—and a stunning headline-when, in July 2002, the Women's Health Initiative announced that it was simply stopping a long-term clinical trial of the combination HRT because of its health risks. Two years later, the WHI stopped a study of estrogen-only HRT—also because of health risks. At the same time, the legendary Nurses' Health Study carried out by the Harvard Medical School confirmed that the combination estrogen-progestin was "more harmful than it was helpful."

What were the effects of these HRT treatments? Except for an improved mood and the reduced risk of osteoporosis-induced bone fracture and colon cancer, women taking the combination treatment could look forward to pretty much the opposite of its promised benefits. Women on this form of HRT suffered more heart attacks, more strokes, more risk of heart disease, and greater risk of breast cancer than women not using the therapy. They also suffered more dry eye, although not as badly as the women in the estrogen-only group. For that group, the finding was that the women were 70 percent more likely to develop dry eyes. Moreover, the longer the women were on estrogen, the greater the risk and the worse the symptoms. The equation was pretty clear: estrogen-and-progesterone combined had some drying effect on the eyes; estrogen alone had a very profound drying effect on the eyes.

The bottom line of these extraordinary studies, while certainly alarming for post-menopausal women in general, was scientifically extremely important. The studies' findings gave rise to further study, observation, and analysis across a range of issues. One of the most interesting of these issues was the estrogen–dry eye link—that is, the finding that estrogen has some effect that results in dry eye.

It should be said that researchers were not universally convinced about the drying effect of the combination estrogen-progestin therapy. It was noted that the study "results" came in the form of questionnaire answers submitted by the study's subjects—not from clinical examination by trained and experienced eye doctors. To many observers, the conclusions drawn from the combination-therapy study warranted further analysis. In addition, there has since been some conflicting evidence that estrogen might offer a protective effect against dry eye. This evidence derives from the observation that there seems to be a rise in the incidence of dry eye in post-menopausal women. As of this writing, however, the weight of the data appears to lean the other way. While the estrogen-progestin findings may constitute a gray area, the findings about dry eye drawn from the estrogen-only study seems conclusive: there is a link between estrogen and dry eye.

A recent study by the National Eye Institute would seem to offer dramatic confirmation of that estrogen–dry eye link. The NEI study focused on women with premature ovarian failure, which occurs in just one percent of women under the age of 40. This unhappy condition effectively produces all the symptoms of the post-menopausal state but at a young age. One of the symptoms experienced by these women is severe dry eye. Indeed, compared to women of their own age, the women afflicted with premature ovarian failure suffer all the discomforts associated with advanced dry eye: blurry vision, eye pain, burning, stinging, grittiness. Again, it would seem that there is a definite link between estrogen and dry eye—at any age.

None of these studies have been able to tell us precisely how the mechanism of the link might work, but that there is a link seems certain. Interestingly, and in a way that complicates the issue, the WHI and Nurses' studies have also showed that other common eye conditions—cataracts, glaucoma, and macular degeneration—are actually improved with the use of HRT.

I've seen evidence of the estrogen connection to dry eye in my own practice as well. Deborah was 27 years old and healthy in every way—except for her complaint of eye discomfort. She had tried the usual over-the-counter drops, but their effect had been no better than temporary. Deborah had no idea what could be causing her dry eye, and it wasn't until I had taken a thorough history that I had a hint about the cause. It turned out that Deborah's symptoms had begun six months before, at precisely the time, as questioning revealed, that she began taking a different kind of oral contraceptive from the one she had been using previously. I had a talk with Deborah's obstetrician, who had prescribed the contraceptives in order to regulate Deborah's irregular periods, and indeed, the switch six months before had been from a pill with a low amount of estrogen to one with a high estrogen content. The obstetrician agreed to switch Deborah's prescription back to a low-estrogen pill; within months, Deborah's dry eye symptoms had simply disappeared.

To all readers, this should serve as a reminder, should one be needed, that oral contraception is powerful medicine; it has been connected to blood clots in the eyes, so it clearly can affect your eyes; and it should only be taken under the careful supervision of your gynecologist. To me, however, the real issue in Deborah's case was that it offered convincing evidence indeed of the link between estrogen and dry eye.

But what is the link? We don't know. We simply have no idea as yet just what the mechanism is or how it works. The theory, however, is that estrogen in some way promotes inflammation of the ocular surface, which, as we know, is now the suspected first cause of dry eye.

The Androgen Connection

By contrast, androgen, the male hormone found in both sexes, appears to suppress inflammation in and around the eyes. In fact, there is now a fairly definitive link between inflammation of the tear-secreting meibomian glands and the decreased production of androgen. The link goes a step further: not only does insufficient androgen potentially cause dry eye, but it is also the case that abundant androgen appears to reduce the risk of dry eye. Somehow, in other words, androgen promotes better functioning of the meibomian glands; it appears to regulate at least the quality if not also the quantity of the oily secretions from the glands, thus playing a role in coating the tear film and preventing it from breaking down and evaporating.

We have evidence for this in the case of those men who, for other health reasons—most notably, a prostate condition—have taken anti-androgen therapy. One result is an increase in these men of dry eye; the tear film simply breaks down faster. Evidence from other studies indicates that the androgen connection is not a matter of quantity of tears; rather, according to these studies, it is the quality of the oily secretions produced by the meibomian glands that is the key factor.

The Bottom Line on Hormones

The bottom line on these two hormones is this: where estrogen evidently stimulates inflammation in the eyes, androgen evidently suppresses it, even though we're not sure how.

What does this mean in practical terms—especially to women in their later, post-menopausal years, a group that is disproportionately afflicted with dry eye? In a sense, it comes down to the volume of hormones present in members of both sexes. Put in the most simplistic terms: while both sexes have both hormones—estrogen and androgen—and while the amount of these hormones declines with age in both sexes, women start out with more estrogen and less androgen, so as the supplies of both decline, it is the extreme paucity of androgen in women that may be decisive in causing and/or exacerbating dry eye. As for men, you seem to be on the protective side of this equation—unless you have a condition that warrants some form of hormone therapy.

There's plenty of evidence to support this theory. For example, a drop in androgen levels occurs not just during menopause but also during pregnancy, during breast-feeding, and during the use of estrogen-containing oral contraceptives, as we saw with Deborah. All of these drops in androgen level have been connected to a concomitant decline in the functioning of the tear-secreting meibomian glands.

Now in addition comes the discovery that women with Sjögren's syndrome are deficient in androgen. In fact, it is today being theorized that androgen deficiency may be a link in other autoimmune diseases—including lupus—and animal studies now underway hint that some use of androgen therapy may be useful for these diseases. Such therapy is certainly in the works for Sjögren's sufferers, and it is also in the pipeline for those afflicted with dry eye.

Hormone Therapy for Dry Eye

The evidence about hormones and dry eye appears to be airtight, although certainly, our understanding of how the connection might work is far from perfect. The jury is still out, at least to some extent, on the precise nature of the estrogen connection, although there is a general consensus that androgen plays a strong role in the development of dry eye—that an androgen deficiency is telling in preventing or suppressing the inflammation that is the first cause of the disorder. Those indications are sufficiently compelling, at any rate, that the development of hormone therapy for dry eye is an idea whose time has come.

As of this writing, at least two groups of researchers are pursuing two different approaches to such therapy. The pharmaceutical giant Allergan, along with a group of scientists from Harvard University, has developed an androgen eye drop that is now in advanced clinical testing. Another group of researchers, from the Aborn Eye Research Center at the New York Eye & Ear Infirmary, has been looking more closely at developing a combination androgen-estrogen hormone eye drop. This initiative is also in advanced clinical testing.

We will have to wait and see which of these therapies is the more effective, but that hormones will play an increasingly important role in the future treatment of dry eye is indisputable. As our understanding of the mechanism of hormone involvement improves—as we come to understand the exact nature of the link between hormones and dry eye—those treatments will only get better, and the future for dry eye patients will only grow brighter.

11

PUNCTAL PLUGS AND OTHER MEANS OF KEEPING THE TEARS IN WITHOUT DRUGS

How about a prescription for dry eye disorder that doesn't use medicine at all? It's not only possible, it's one of the most effective solutions in the ophthalmologist's toolkit.

Just ask Betsy. By the time she came to see me, this contact-lens wearer had been through a battery of tests wisely prescribed by her eye doctor in response to her complaint of cloudy central vision. After a visual field test revealed a central defect in the eye, Betsy's doctor sent her for a CT scan that showed nothing, an MRI that showed nothing, and a range of blood tests that showed nothing. Three different eye doctors then conferred on the results—and all agreed there was no discernible cause for her cloudy central vision. That was when she was referred to me.

When I entered the examining room, I confronted an attractive 37-year-old with rather large, prominent eyes. That raised my antennae at once; I immediately suspected dryness related to exposure of the eye and proceeded to perform my Tear Normalization Test, the TNT, applying a drop of plain old over-the-counter tear solution in each eye. "Wow!" was Betsy's response. "What did you just do? I can see crystal clear!"

Her reaction confirmed my diagnosis: a dry eye surface. After all, her eyes were not inflamed nor swollen. So it wasn't that her lacrimal glands were functioning poorly; it was just that they weren't producing sufficient tears to keep her eye surface moist, especially given the bulging of her eyes. The bulging, by the way, was due to natural genetic causes in Betsy's case—she was just born with nice big eyes—and not to surgery, which is another common reason for exposure. Either way, the fact that with the right tear film she could see perfectly made it clear that surface dryness was the problem. She needed more tears.

In Betsy's case, given her medical situation—insufficient tear production—and her adventurous personality, we determined that the simplest and most effective solution would be punctal plugs. Now "punctal plugs" is not a very pretty-sounding phrase, but they can be a lovely alternative to medicines or over-the-counter drops, and the relief they bring to dry eye sufferers can be downright beautiful.

Simply put, punctal plugs are very, very tiny rods that can be inserted into the very, very tiny holes in the upper and/or lower eyelid. You've seen those holes; they're right in the inside corner of the eye, near the nose. The plugs are about the size of an eye-

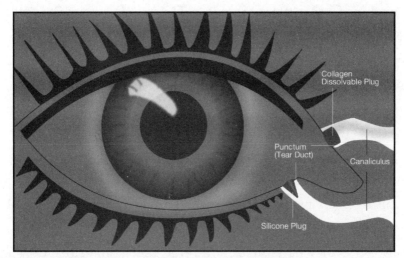

Figure 11: *Location of silicone or collagen punctal plug implants*

lash: 0.2 to 0.5 millimeters wide and less than two millimeters in length. To get an idea of what those measurements mean, consider that you can fit nearly 18 millimeters on a U.S. dime.

The technology of the plugs is pretty simple: the idea is to keep the eyes moist by plugging up the holes through which the tears might drain. Betsy, for example, would compensate for her deficient tear production by simply keeping more tears in her eyes—or rather, by having the punctal plugs keep more tears in her eyes.

Simple it may be, but it works. What's more, inserting the plugs is easy, absolutely painless, and takes less than five seconds to do. There are three types of punctal plugs, giving three options for treatment.

Collagen plugs. Collagen plugs connect to a tube that channels the tears to a sac inside the nose, from which the tears exit through an opening in the back of the nose. This whole apparatus is called the naso-lacrimal drainage system, and by plugging up the system with the collagen plug, you simply keep the tears from exiting through the canal—and keep the eyes moist.

Collagen plugs are temporary, however—by design. (They can also fall out—not by design—either through the nose or through the eye, although patients are rarely aware of it.) They come in two varieties–those meant to last a few days and those meant to last a few months. That makes the collagen plugs the perfect starter kit for people who don't like the whole idea of plugs. Since they have virtually no side effects, and since they are made of a "natural" substance found in the body, collagen, they can serve as an initial tryout that lets patients see if blocking the drainage duct helps them. If they don't help, the entire impact has been only temporary, and no harm has been done; doctor and patient will simply need to seek another kind of therapy. If the collagen plugs do help, it might be a signal to move on to silicone plugs, which offer permanent relief.

Silicone plugs. Silicone plugs are slightly larger than the collagen but are meant to last forever. Each is shaped like an arrow, with a pointed head and a capped distal end. Once it's inserted, the cap holds the plug in place, and the plug holds the tears in the eye. And while a doctor can see the cap, it is only visible to the patient when he or she averts the eyelid and looks for it under strong light; the wider public of family and friends won't notice it at all.

If there's a downside to the silicone plugs, it is that some 10 to 15 percent of wearers feel the plug, and that about half of the plugs inserted do fall out after a couple of years. For those that can wear them comfortably and keep them, however, they could mean an end to artificial tears or just about any other treatment. You need do nothing at all; just let the plugs hold in your tears so that there's an excess of them, keeping your eyes nice and moist.

That's what happened with Betsy. I advised her to stop using her contact lenses except on very rare occasions, and I inserted the silicone plugs. That was four years ago. The plugs are still there and still working beautifully. Betsy sees well, uses her lenses sparingly, has no irritation, no dryness, no complaints— and plenty of tears.

Buried plugs. Finally, the third type of punctal plug is a category I call the "buried plug." This type of plug is literally pushed into that channel between eyelid and nose such that no part of it sticks out; it cannot be detected at all. Since buried plugs don't protrude in any way, wearers never have the sense that there's a foreign body in the eye, as some 10 percent to 15 percent of other punctal plug wearers do.

There are four types of buried plugs, all made from different materials. The four types are the Smart Plug, made of an acrylic material; the Form Fit plug by Oasis Medical, made of a hydrogel; Alcon's Tears Naturale, made of silicone; and a new entry by FCI Ophthalmic, also made of silicone. All are designed to shrink in length but expand in width to fill up the naso-lacrimal canal. That means, however, that to remove the plugs, it takes either an almost surgical procedure to pluck them out or that you must irrigate the canal and wash the plugs into the nose—versus the five-second removal of the silicone plugs, for example.

What dampens my enthusiasm for the buried plugs, however, is that I can't see them. I want to be able to see the plugs so I know they're there and doing their job. Once they're beneath the punctum and buried inside the canal, I'm at a loss to know whether or not they're having an effect.

Still, punctal plugs offer a range of options to meet varied medical and comfort needs. They are an alternative to drugs that is attractive to many—a quick fix with a wow-factor benefit and virtually no adverse side effects. In the eyes of many of my patients—and yes, I mean to use just those words—punctal plugs are nothing short of a miracle.

Cautery

The truth is, however, that there are some people who just cannot bear having a foreign object in their eyes. And there are others–automatic eye-rubbers, for example—who can't seem to hold punctal plugs in place; they like the effect the plugs produce, but they don't like their frequent trips to the eye doctor's office to have new ones put in.

But once we know that blocking the ducts works for treating the dry eye, there's an alternative to punctal plugs that produces the same effect: cauterizing the punctum.

The procedure is simple and quick and can be performed easily in the doctor's office. A minute amount of local anesthetic is applied right next to the punctum's opening. Either a heating probe or a laser can be used for the procedure itself; I prefer the probe. I simply place the needle-like probe in the hole and push a button to release heat from the tip of the needle. The heat zaps the tissue, and this creates a tiny scar that will block the opening and seal it off. As with punctal plugs, sealing off the ducts just keeps more tears in the eye.

One category of patients for whom cautery works well is Asian patients. The anatomy of the Asian eye is such that in many people—including a patient I recently treated—the eyelids curl inwards a bit. My patient, who suffered from a serious case of dry eye, had had punctal plugs installed repeatedly by different doctors but had never found them comfortable. In her case, as in the case of many Asians, the structure of the eyelid forced the plug to rub up against the eyeball, causing the discomfort. She wasn't even willing to try buried plugs, so instead, I performed cautery. It worked well—both for her comfort level and for treating her dry eye.

Boston Scleral Lens

The Boston scleral lens is a prosthetic device the size of a quarter that is placed over the eye like a contact lens. Highly oxygen-permeable, the scleral lens rests on the insensitive white tissue of the eye—the sclera—and holds a reservoir of artificial tears over the cornea. It thus acts as a liquid bandage for the eye.

The Boston scleral lens has proven to be effective in many patients with severe and incapacitating dry eyes who have reached a dead end in other dry eye treatments. It can be an alternative for corneal transplant surgery or tarsorrhaphy.

Currently, the lenses are only being fitted at the Boston Foundation for Sight, where the technology was developed, and you need a referral from your eye doctor.

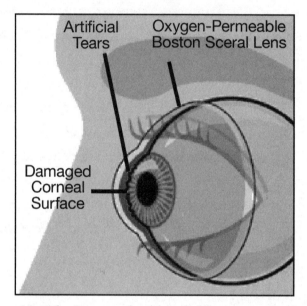

Figure 12: *The Boston scleral lens holds a reservoir of artificial tears over the cornea*

1 2

SURGICAL INTERVENTION

Surgery is typically the intervention of last resort for dealing with the disorders of the ocular surface. Rightly so. Since surgery is the most aggressive therapy there is, logic alone dictates that other interventions should be tried first. In addition, no surgical procedure, despite its aggressive character, can guarantee 100 percent success. It is always wiser, therefore, to save surgery till it is absolutely necessary or till the weight of the evidence makes it the single most effective possible therapy.

Of course, there are such situations that reach that point of necessity. And to deal with them, there is a wide and growing range of surgical options. Those options may be thought of as falling into any of three categories: eyelid-altering procedures, surgical interventions on the eye surface, and some fairly experimental procedures focusing on the tear-secreting glands.

Eyelid-Altering Procedures

Since dryness often derives from having too much exposed ocular surface for the amount of tears available, simply reducing the area of the eye surface that is exposed can alleviate the dryness. And one way to do that is by altering the eyelids.

There are a number of techniques for doing this. Tarsorrhaphy was mentioned in the previous chapter; it's a simple procedure in which the outer edges of the upper and lower eyelids are literally sewn together very slightly. Look in a mirror as you take your thumb and index finger of one hand and gently squeeze the outer edges of your eyelids together. You can see how the size of the opening is reduced, thus reducing the area of exposed ocular surface and keeping more of the surface lubricated. That's exactly what a tarsorrhaphy does.

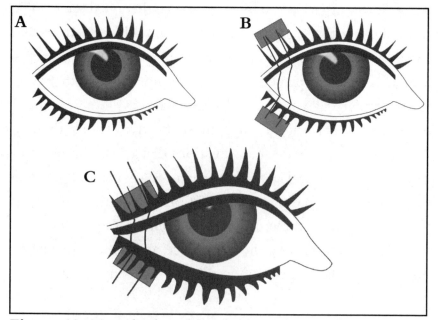

Figure 13: *Tarsorrhaphy reduces the exposed eye surface area*

The extent of the closure in tarsorrhaphy will depend on the severity of the situation. One or two sutures applied in the doctor's office usually suffice for a mild condition, but some situations may require more than that, and an operating room setting might be preferable. In either case, only a local anesthetic is required.

A patient I'll call Diana represents a not uncommon case where a tarsorrhaphy made a real difference. At age 50, Diana had recently suffered a painful episode of Bell's palsy, one effect of which is the weakening of the seventh cranial nerve, the very nerve responsible for closing the eyelids. Bell's palsy sufferers are therefore typically at risk of blinking only incompletely during the day and of sleeping with the eyes slightly open so that the lower part of the eye tends to dry out pretty badly.

That was certainly the case with Diana. Her eyes were causing her discomfort, and her vision was blurry by the time her internist referred her to me. My examination found relatively severe dryness of Diana's ocular surface as well as substantial thinning of her cornea. I considered her situation fairly risky; it was conceivable that the cornea might rupture, with consequences as potentially disastrous as the loss of the eye. Aggressive treatment was certainly called for, and we began with a rigorous course of ointments and drops as well as the use of punctal plugs. When none of these therapies stopped the thinning of the corneal layer, it was time to do a tarsorrhaphy.

But Bell's palsy is a condition that typically resolves over time, so in Diana's case, the procedure was a temporary tarsorrhaphy. The severity of her dryness called for a tarsorrhaphy that was certainly somewhat disfiguring, but it worked: the tear-secreting glands didn't have to work quite so hard to cover Diana's eyes with the appropriate amount of a healthy, stable tear film.

About a month after the procedure, the palsy improved, and Diana's seventh nerve began to function better. It was then relatively easy to remove the sutures and go back to a regimen of ointments, drops, and plugs—cosmetically much more pleasing—until the surface of the eye regained its structural integrity.

Sometimes, especially in cases of severe chronic conditions, a permanent tarsorrhaphy is required. This is a more complex procedure in which the surgeon literally scrapes off surface layers of the eyelids so that the areas of the upper and lower lids that are to be connected are deliberately made raw surfaces. Once they are sewn together, the two raw surfaces begin to heal; in doing so, they scar, and the scarring forms a tight seal that keeps the connection permanent.

Another option among eyelid-altering procedures is called a cisternoplasty. In this procedure, the outside corner of the eye is formed into a small pocket that serves as a reservoir of tears.

Finally, a quasi-surgical procedure that alters the eyelids is to inject Botox into the lid. Just as Botox smoothes out facial wrinkles, it effectively weakens the upper eyelid muscle till it droops, thus decreasing the exposed surface area of the eye. And just as in the use of Botox for cosmetic reasons, the effects of this induced droopiness are also temporary.

Stem Cell Transplants

Jim was 35 and had been prescribed a routine oral antibiotic for what he and his doctor thought was a routine ear infection. But

Jim's reaction to the medication was devastating: he developed a full body rash, ulcerations appeared in and around his mouth, and his eyes became inflamed and scarred. By the time he came to my office, the ocular surface had broken down sufficiently that Jim's vision had been substantially affected. At first, we tried a variety of topical therapies three times a week. But the results were inadequate, so we made the decision to perform a stem cell transplant procedure.

Stem cells are of course vital for providing replacement cells throughout the body, and an adequate stem cell population is essential to a healthy ocular surface. You'll find this population just at the point where the cornea meets the white of the eye, called the sclera. Various conditions can reduce this population of stem cells or kill them off. Accidents—like having acid or lye splatter into the eye—can certainly cause such results. But so can the chronic use of contact lenses. One of the most horrific causes of stem cell deficiency or death is the life-threatening Stevens Johnson syndrome, mentioned back in Chapter 2, an extremely severe reaction to over-the-counter or prescription drugs. In Stevens Johnson sufferers, severe dry eye disorder typically results from the loss of goblet cells, the scarring of the glands, and the extreme irregularities in the skin surface of the eye. Serious loss of vision is often a consequence.

This was in fact what had happened to Jim, and since both his eyes were affected by his reaction to the antibiotic, we had to look elsewhere for a stem cell source. One of the places we might normally look is to an eye bank that preserves the eyes donated through living wills—or, in some states, designated for donation on the backs of drivers' licenses. Since there's virtually no chance of a genetic match with such donors, the patient typically has to take oral steroids and other immuno-suppressants for some time to ensure that the transplanted cells are not rejected. Fortunately, however, in Jim's case, his brother was eager to volunteer some of his own ocular stem cells—blood relatives offer a good chance of a match—and I was able to cut off a skin layer from the brother and simply sew it into place in Jim's eyes, with highly successful results. An even more promising possibility coming to the fore as of this writing involves taking a piece of tissue from the patient's inner cheek and sending it to a lab where it grows into a sheet of stem cells that can be transplanted weeks later. There's no worry at all about a match or about rejection in such a situation because it comes from your own body.

Stem cell transplants are not the first line of defense when there is a stem cell deficiency, but they represent a most effective therapy when needed. The fresh stem cells almost literally polish

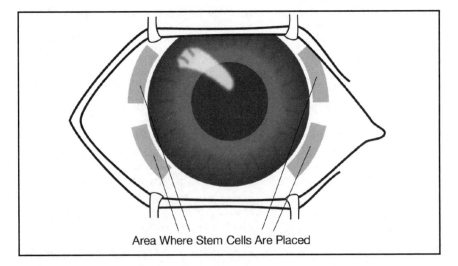

Area Where Stem Cells Are Placed

Figure 14: *Location where stem cells are transplanted*

the ocular surface; they restore the health and structural sound-ness of the eye's skin, and this makes dryness far easier to manage.

But stem cells aren't the only things that can be surgically transplanted to deal with dysfunctional tear film. Eye banks now also store sheets of amniotic membrane—yes, the same membrane that forms the innermost layer of the placenta—for use in all sorts of reconstructive surgery. As a way to restore the soundness or smoothness of the eye's surface, performing an amniotic membrane transplant is like putting down a starting fertilizer on your lawn; the skin that grows over the transplanted membrane will come in strong.

Other Eye Surface Surgeries
Think of a running brook, the water bubbling downstream swiftly with that telltale gurgling sound. Now picture a large boulder in mid-stream, and see how the water parts as it comes up against the boulder, streaming around it to either side. As a result, the top of the boulder stays dry, and the "back" of the boulder, its downstream face, also gets no lubrication from the oncoming stream.

The same thing can happen in the eye, where any wrinkling of the surface or protuberance or even stretching of the surface skin breaks up the tear film the way a boulder breaks up a run-ning brook. Nothing beyond the protruding piece of the surface gets properly lubricated, and the protrusion itself stays dry.

All sorts of things can cause this state of affairs, which, when it occurs over the white of the eye is called conjunctivochalasis, meaning a redundancy or swelling of the conjunctiva. A chronic health condition, heredity, or even aging can inflame and/or impair the ocular surface. As with badly wrinkled or sagging skin, this redundant skin on the eye surface usually sticks out a bit, disrupting what ought to be smooth and virtually spherical surface. In fact, some patients with this condition complain of a bulge or blister or small cyst growing on their eye. This is quite a common development, and over time, as you might imagine, the redundancy will dry out considerably, causing all the irritations and discomforts of dry eye syndrome.

Surgery simply cuts the redundancy out of the eye. The surgeon excises the excess skin, then sews the edges of the surface back together for a tighter fit—somewhat the way a plastic surgeon tightens wrinkled facial skin. It is a very simple procedure that uses absorbable sutures so that only one trip to the operating room is required. And of course, the procedure needs just a local anesthetic.

A similar procedure will work any time an irregular surface causes symptoms that don't respond to other treatments— whether the irregularity is structural or due to an infection or scar or perhaps caused by a contact lens–related ulcer. The idea is simply to even out the surface so that the tear film won't face any obstacles as it tries to maintain a smooth, consistent surface.

Kevin was 45, and over the previous year had suffered four attacks of sharp eye pain, sharp enough to wake him in the night. By the time he came to see me, he had tried a range of drops and salves with no success, was suffering chronic dryness, and the quality of his vision had deteriorated to the point where he could not see distance well at all. After examining Kevin, I diagnosed a condition called map-dot-fingerprint dystrophy. It's an unusual name, but the condition is actually fairly common. The name derives from the appearance of the ocular surface through the slit lamp: it has outlines that look like continents on a map, may have clusters of dots, or will exhibit concentric lines that resemble fingerprints. Map-dot-fingerprint dystrophy causes the recurrent bouts of corneal erosion that had caused Kevin such pain in the night, and the ocular surface tends not to heal correctly. Since typical treatments were not working, and since Kevin's dry eye disorder was severe, I decided to use laser surgery to solve the problem.

In the procedure I devised for Kevin, I scraped the irregular skin off his cornea and, once that was done, used a laser to surgically create his prescription for nearsightedness, just as in PRK or LASIK surgery. The fact is that the surface skin would grow back over the cornea in any event once the irregular, blurry skin has been scraped off; lasering in the prescription not only corrected Kevin's vision but also created a stickier surface so that the new skin would seal down better. Result? Kevin was free of the mildly opaque skin and poorly adhering that was causing his blurry vision, pain, and dryness; he did not need to wear eyeglasses; and, as an extra bonus, his medical insurance covered the entire procedure!—an unusual occurrence as PRK and LASIK procedures are typically not covered.

Altering the Tear-Secreting Glands

A number of new procedures, some of which sound almost fanciful, are today focusing on altering the tear-secreting glands themselves. Though still very much in the experimental stage—and being pursued mostly outside the United States—there may indeed be something to the idea behind these attempts.

One idea is to transplant some of the submandibular gland, the gland under the jawbone, to a point underneath the eyelids. The point here is simply to replace tear-secreting glands that are not functioning well—those in the eyelid—with one that does function well. Odd though it sounds, the transplant reportedly works.

Even odder, however, is a procedure that implants a reservoir in the belly cavity; a tube carries a constant flow of "tears" all the way up to the eyes. Unfortunately, the reservoir needs to be replaced every 40 days, which would seem to mitigate against the practicality of this solution.

And going beyond odd to comical is a procedure that focuses on the parotid gland, the gland in front of the ear that is responsible for secreting saliva in the mouth via a tube from the ear to the inside of the mouth. In the procedure, the ear-to-mouth tube is redirected to the lower eyelid; even though saliva is not quite the composition of tear film, it is not far off, and the extra moisture does help lubricate the eye.

The procedure produces an unfortunate side effect, however: patients report that when they even think about eating their favorite food, their eyes tear up excessively; in effect, the eyes start salivating!

Yet no matter how comical some of these experiments may sound, the impulse behind them is not to be taken lightly. For they are evidence that both doctors and patients are on the lookout for new therapies and original solutions that can treat, manage, and alleviate the real suffering caused by dysfunctional tear film syndrome and the disorders of dry eye.

PART FOUR

FINDING THE DRY EYE THERAPY THAT WORKS FOR YOU

Now that you have a good idea of the broad range of lifestyle and environmental adjustments, medications, and other options that can relieve your dry eyes, how do you put it all together into a therapy that works for you?

Part Four puts everything we've learned so far together for you, describing likely courses of treatment for various dry eye conditions and levels of intensity.

In Chapter 13, you can identify your "treatment personality" to ensure that you choose the approach you are most comfortable and therefore most likely to stick with—always the biggest challenge in treating a chronic condition like dry eye.

Finally, Chapter 14 looks at the state of dry eye today in both the medical community and in public consciousness and peers into the future of dry eye research and relief. There are a number of exciting possibilities in the pipeline for dry eye treatment, including hormone-based approaches and anti-inflammatory medications. We look forward to the time when there is not a dry eye in the house.

13

FOUR THERAPEUTIC APPROACHES TO DRY EYES

Now that you've learned the various kinds of medications that might be used for dry eye, as well as the environmental and nutritional adjustments that can help alleviate the symptoms of the disorder, you pretty much know the tools of the eye doctor's trade when it comes to treating the dysfunction. So what might you or any dry eye sufferer expect in the way of a therapeutic program that will both bring a measure of relief today and keep the worst effects of the disorder at bay?

First of all, it's important to state a proposition that is about as basic to the physician's credo as the Hippocratic Oath—that is, that every patient is unique and must be treated on an absolutely individual basis. Any course of treatment prescribed will depend on the particular stage of the disorder at which the patient has arrived, the intensity of the disorder, and the specific symptoms it is causing, as well as on the individual's history, allergies, age, other health conditions, if any, and general state of well-being.

It's also essential for patients themselves to participate in both understanding the cause of their dry eye and defining the treatment. In fact, in my view, if there is one thing that is absolutely key to the successful treatment of the disorder that I've been able to achieve with my patients, it's jut that: I've achieved the success with my patients. Together, we take a detailed history. Together, we do the detective work so necessary for determining the root cause of the dry eye. Together, we figure out a course of treatment that can work. Then I prescribe and recommend, the patient applies and executes, and we continue to meet, monitor, and consult on progress.

Obviously, we cannot do that in this book. But if I cannot prescribe in these pages, I can describe the typical courses of treatment for restoring eye health to dry eye sufferers. I break down those courses of treatment into six, corresponding to what are six categories of patient who come to me for relief from their dry eye disorder:

1. **First-Timers**—individuals who for the first time worry that "something is up" with their eyes. Perhaps they feel a mild dryness, or perhaps they simply wonder why they need a new eyeglass prescription every two years, or perhaps they just don't want to suffer the same annoying symptoms their parents suffered with their eyes. This group is more curious than concerned.

2. **The Stymied**—individuals who are frustrated that their over-the-counter artificial tears don't seem to be helping.

This group is seeking more relief than they're getting with their current treatment.

3. **Been There/Done That**—individuals who come to my office with a list of the medications they've taken and sample bottles of the drops that haven't worked. These people are sure they have done everything possible for the disorder; they're pretty fed up and not too hopeful.

4. **The All-Naturals**—individuals who do not trust pharmaceutical drugs and who may not really like seeking medical help from MDs. These folks are at the end of their rope, but there are rules about what they will and will not do in terms of treatment.

5. **The Pre-Surgicals**—individuals who are about to have cataract surgery, plastic surgery, or any form of eye surgery and have been referred by their surgeons. These patients have been assured that their surgery will be more successful and their recovery easier if they are first treated with eyelid-cleansing and other restoring procedures.

6. **The Just-Fix-It Crowd**—individuals who want the most convenient regimen possible for their dry eye. They don't want to use drops, do treatments at home, or even know what's wrong; they just want it fixed.

Charting Your Own Course of Treatment

With a good medical history, such as the one in Chapter 3, and with all that you've learned about tear film dysfunction in the preceding pages, you should be able to determine pretty precisely which category you're in. Keep in mind that the courses of treatment I'm about to describe are typical; that doesn't necessarily mean any particular course is right for you. But if the course of treatment you're on now is markedly different from the ones I describe, you might want to discuss the discrepancy with your doctor.

It's important to try each course of treatment for at least 14 days. Experience has shown that the two-week mark is a good time to re-assess; 14 days give the treatment a chance to work, and the end of the two-week period is a good time to call a halt, catch your breath, and check the direction of your forward motion. If there's no improvement in the dry eye symptoms after two weeks, that might be the signal to try something else; if there is improvement, it might be a good idea to adjust dosage or add or subtract a healing factor in the course of treatment.

Let's take them category by category:

First-Timers. Since the issue here is "something wrong" or an early diagnosis of dry eye or prevention, it's best to proceed conservatively, initiating the most basic course of treatment first. I would therefore prescribe over-the-counter preservative-free tear drops, which I recommend the patient chill in the refrigerator and keep chilled in the carrier sack. For reasons of convenience and to keep expenses down, I would certainly suggest the patient buy those tears with disappearing preservative. For patients I suspect have lagophthalmos, I would also recommend a nighttime ointment. In addition to these medications, I would prescribe the Home Eye Spa treatment for eyelid hygiene.

It's also important for first-timers to begin the detective work toward determining the root cause of their dryness. They should certainly start with the questionnaire in Chapter 5 and should monitor also how their eyes respond to various irritants: smoke, spicy-hot aromas, perfumes, cold air, hot air, and the like. The question is simple: where were you and what were you doing when your eyes felt bad, and where were you and what were you doing when your eyes felt particularly good? In response to their detective work, first-timers should make whatever environmental adjustments they can.

In addition, first-timers should be aware of the nutritional component of their disorder; they might try avoiding foods that cause inflammation, and they might want to start beefing up their intake of omega-3 fatty acids as a preventive measure at least.

To contact lens wearers, I would suggest that they reduce the amount of time they wear their lenses or that they change from the long-wearing type of lens to a type that is cleaned and "refreshed" more frequently.

The Stymied. If these folks have not done all the things I've prescribed for first-timers, their first step should be to do so—they need to go right back to basics. This will enable them, by a careful process of elimination, to get rid of the tears and ointments that don't work for them—although I recommend they keep cold tears on hand to soothe eyes that are particularly inflamed or itchy. In addition, they should begin to make the Home Eye Spa treatment a habit and should undertake the environmental and nutritional adjustments that can make such a substantial difference. The contact lens wearers among them should take special care in cleaning their lenses.

But the main treatment change I would recommend for the stymied would be either a combination of Restasis and Lotemax or the use of punctal plugs—both of which require a prescription and both of which are covered by insurance. Which solution is best? The answer may rest more with the patient's personal desires than with science. Some individuals recoil from the idea of punctal plugs, while others would far rather have a one-shot procedure than a course of medicines. Obviously, the solution that the patient will faithfully apply is the treatment to choose.

The Lotemax-Restasis solution does require the patient to be conscientious in applying the medications. Twice a day, he or she will apply the Lotemax first, then the Restasis ten minutes later. A mild steroid, the Lotemax offers instant relief and thus eases patients through the initial stages of Restasis till its considerable benefits kick in. Once that happens—and it typically takes a few weeks—the Lotemax, which serves only as a palliative, may be discontinued as the patients persist with the Restasis.

The punctal plug solution, by contrast, requires a procedure in the doctor's office. At first, the plugs should be applied to the lower eyelid only. If that works, fine; if not, the plugs may be applied to the upper eyelids as well in a second procedure.

I would further recommend that any contact lens wearers in this group switch to the daily disposable lenses, and I would urge all patients in the stymied category to take Dry-Vites for the benefits of omega-3 fatty acids in its fish oil/flaxseed oil combination—unless they already take a preferred brand of fish oil.

Been There/Done That. Actually, the first thing I urge from these people is patience. It's important to know not just what they've tried but how they have tried it. For example, a patient may claim to have "tried Restasis but it didn't work." I would want to know how long that trial lasted: did the patient really persist with the Restasis despite some initial discomfort? Did the patient's doctor explain that the discomfort from Restasis might last for a few weeks before its benefits were felt? Was any palliative offered? If the answer to any or all of these questions was no, the patient cannot be said to have failed treatment; rather, he simply didn't give the medicine enough of a chance to succeed.

So for this category of patients as well, it may be advisable to go back to basics and do the first-timer regimen—the Home Eye Spa treatment, the detective work, the environmental monitoring and adjustments. But once it's been determined that these folks really have "tried everything," the next step would be to figure out the source of their problem. Then, depending on the first cause, I might prescribe oral tetracycline to address blepharitis or meibomian gland dysfunction—especially if the patient shows signs of rosacea; the antibiotic tetracycline kills off the bacteria and helps fight the inflammation. Or a prescription for autologous serum drops might help repair the ocular surface, and I might also prescribe either punctal plugs for both upper and lower eyelids or punctal cauterization, which "plugs" the punctal ducts with heat. These patients might also be likely candidates for clinical trials, and I would work with the patient to identify the right clinical trial for his or her particular case.

At the same time, I would ask the patient to stop using contact lenses altogether. I would suggest the use of tranquileyes at night and moisture chamber goggles—i.e., motorcycle glasses—during the day. In addition to the patient's own performance of the Home Eye Spa treatment, these individuals would benefit from the special version of the Eye Spa treatment performed in my office. This treatment consists of eyelid-cleansing, use of heat, expressing of the gland contents, cooling, and lymph draining via acupressure. It is a very thorough cleaning and immensely soothing as well.

In those cases where there might be risk of vision loss among the individuals in this category, a surgical procedure might be prescribed. Tarsorrhaphy is one such procedure, as we learned in Chapter 11; in this eyelid-altering procedure, the outer edges of the eyelids are closed very slightly in order to reduce the eye opening and thus keep more of the ocular surface lubricated.

The All-Naturals. So much of the therapy for dry eye disorder is all-natural, and I would recommend all of it to this category of patients. Certainly, they should use the chilled preservative-free eye drops as needed, should take Dry-Vites daily, could sleep in tranquileyes, and could make regular use of moisture chamber goggles and Soothers.

Even more fundamentally, these patients should do the environmental and nutritional detective work that can help them focus in on those objects and situations that may be exacerbating their condition—and of course they should adjust their environment and nutrition accordingly. Humidifiers in the home are certainly a recommendation in this regard.

In addition, the all-naturals individuals should be conscientious about performing the Home Eye Spa treatment, and I also recommend that they come in for the office eyelid hygiene treatment on a regular basis.

The Pre-Surgicals. My partner in my New York practice, Dr. Mark Speaker, authored the breakthrough paper demonstrating that cleaning the eyelids prior to surgery reduced the chances of infection. Thanks to Mark, eyelid-cleaning is now standard pre-surgical prep before any eye surgery.

The cleaning itself should be started a week before the surgery, accompanied by a course of tetracyclines to further rid the eyelid of any bacteria. Two days before the surgery, I recommend the use of topical antibiotic eye drops—like Vigamox from Alcon or Zymar from Allergan—four times a day. This really prevents any excess bacteria and further reduces the chances of infection.

Many doctors now also recommend that their pre-surgical patients start on Restasis a month before surgery, and I certainly concur with this recommendation—especially for patients about to undergo LASIK surgery, which can be a cause of dryness that may take as much as five years to overcome. The use of Restasis twice a day for a full month before the procedure, however, can sharpen the post-operative visual acuity and reduce the symptoms of the dryness. Patients should stop taking the Restasis two days before the procedure and start it up again a week after the procedure, continuing with it for several months, then re-assessing the situation with their doctor.

The Just-Fix-It Crowd. For this category of patients, who simply "don't want to be bothered" applying drops or doing home treatments, there are some simple recommendations. First, after a careful cleansing of the eyelids, these patients can benefit from punctal plugs or cauterization to close up the punctal ducts. Since they are unwilling to perform the full Home Eye Spa treatment, I would urge them to at least stay a few extra seconds in the shower to gently massage the edges of their eyelids with a finger. They should supplement this meager cleansing with in-office eyelid hygiene treatments on a regular basis.

I also urge these patients to wear tranquileyes when they sleep and to buy a humidifier for the bedroom and possibly one for their living room. After all, all they have to do is plug it in and turn it on.

Follow whichever of these courses of therapy is appropriate for your category of dry eye disorder—and your personality—and you should see real progress after the initial two weeks. My advice at that point? Continue what works, and drop what doesn't. It's as good a prescription for eye health as any I know.

1 4

FUTURE TRENDS AND
RESEARCH

What is the state of dry eye in the United States today in terms of sufferers and potential sufferers, diagnosis, and treatment? My vantage on this question is perhaps unique, for while there are many doctors researching dry eye, I do not at this time know of any other clinical ophthalmologist specializing exclusively in its treatment besides myself. The view is limited nonetheless by what remains a low level of awareness of dry eye on the part of the general public—even though for today's eye doctors, both ophthalmologists and optometrists, the biggest complaint among their patients is symptoms of dry eye.

Yet perhaps the most compelling trend in the picture of dry eye today is the rising tide of awareness—essential not only to the effective treatment of dry eye but to its potential prevention. For this rising tide, I think we must thank above all the Baby

Boomer generation, with its vaunted refusal to go gently into the aging process. As the Boomers enter their 60s, and as many of them begin to feel the effects of dry eye symptoms, they are making themselves heard on the subject—and are demanding solutions and results.

We must also thank the pharmaceutical industry, which has heard the Boomers—and others—loud and clear, and which is responding to what is surely a growing market need. That response has filled drugstore shelves with dry eye products and is filling television screens with commercials for these products, with the result that more and more of the general public is at least familiar with the phrase "dry eye," and more of those becoming aware of the name are finding that it resonates with symptoms they feel.

Another place where awareness of dry eye is on the rise is in medical training. My generation of ophthalmologists could go through medical school and a residency program rarely hearing the term "dry eye," as I did. And for the most part, ophthalmology is still seen as a surgical field and optometry as the realm of experts on glasses and contact lens fitting. But more and more often today, discussion of dry eye at least finds its way into the classroom or receives a mention in on-the-job training. And there is some evidence—which is very gratifying to see—that alternative ways of looking at the health of the eye and alternative methods of treating the eye are gathering speed in the medical profession.

Another arena of awareness and information-sharing is that ubiquitous force for change in all our lives, the Internet. Chat rooms serve as support groups that have created a veritable fraternity of dry eye sufferers. Across wired and wireless networks, they share experiences of suffering, and they no doubt take comfort from the sense that they are not alone in their suffering and discomfort. But they also share tips on what has worked and not worked for them; they share ideas; they reach out to one another in ways not possible before, and their information and ideas stretch to people in places where medical care is not always easily accessible. They may well stir the pot of new initiatives in both diagnosis and treatment; and they are certainly spreading awareness of their disease.

Dry Eye and Associated Conditions

As gratifying as this rise in awareness level, however, at least from my point of view as a physician, is the increasing sense of connectedness with dry eye among those doctors who treat associated conditions and those foundations that promote research and disseminate information about the conditions. In fact, I believe it is incumbent upon doctors to make appropriate referrals when they note a condition beyond their specialty. If my dry eye patient has joint pain, for example, I'll refer him to a rheumatologist. Similarly, if a primary care physician treating a patient for a thyroid condition hears that patient complain of eye irritation, he will (one hopes) refer the patient to an eye doctor. For the interconnectedness among conditions means that treating, or not treating, one will certainly affect the other.

To take just one example, it is essential for the doctors who treat diabetics to be aware of the ways in which decreased or altered sensation on the surface of these patients' eyes can allow damage to the ocular surface to go virtually unnoticed. If a patient feels no symptoms—if he or she is effectively asymptomatic—then it is up to the examining physician to search for other signs of disease. The greater the connectedness between dry eye and diabetes foundations, the greater the networking among doctors treating patients with these connected conditions, the more effectively patients will be served and salved. And that is happening increasingly.

It is happening with Sjögren's Syndrome, the chronic, inflammatory, autoimmune disorder characterized primarily by dry mouth and dry eye. It is happening with the terrible afflictions of Stevens-Johnson Syndrome, afflictions resulting from a severe allergic reaction to medication, even routine medication. A range of foundations and specialists serving these syndromes is now far more aware of the complications that dry eye can present in their patients; as a result, these patients may be able to look forward to relief for their dry eye symptoms at least.

But this networking is also occurring in the area of gynecology, for peri-menopausal women seem at particular risk for dry eye as they begin to go through the inevitable hormonal changes. It makes sense, therefore, that women's health experts are now adding dry eye to the list of things to watch for at this stage of life.

It also makes sense that eye doctors and plastic surgeons are increasingly aware of the post-surgical potential for dry eye disorders—and are increasingly open to considering non-invasive treatments for these disorders.

I would wish for a similar increase in awareness among those who treat allergy sufferers and among the allergy sufferers themselves, for the connection between allergy and dry eye offers a major diagnostic challenge to both allergists and ophthalmologists. As we have seen, the symptoms of both allergy and dry eye present in similar ways, and while a patient might have allergy only or dry eye only, he or she will most often have a bit of both. The diagnostic challenge that represents is exacerbated by the treatment challenge, for treating the allergy may worsen the dry eye, while the opposite is also true: treating the dry eye might worsen the allergy. For these reasons, an exacting history—such as I've modeled in Chapter 3—as well as a detailed examination are of critical importance.

I would hope also for greater awareness of the potential for dry eye among those who prescribe contact lenses—and among those who wear them. My suspicion about the increase we're now seeing in dry eye among longtime lens wearers is that people are beginning lens wear at much earlier ages than ever before. Where previous generations typically started wearing contacts in their late teens at the very earliest, today we see children of eight, nine, and ten sporting them. Placing such foreign objects on the ocular surface while the eye is still in its growing stage might conceivably be affecting the overall, long-term health of the eye. Moreover, these children will be wearing lenses for a very long time—well into adulthood and old age, and that longevity itself may create dry eye. In addition, the trend toward the use of cosmetic lenses of every variety— colored, tinted, image, even lenses emblazoned with the team logo!—is unsettling, not just for the idea of looking into some-one's eyes and seeing Go Mets!, but also because such lenses are obviously more toxic than the traditional "plain" variety.

The point is that we do not really know the long-term impact of cosmetic lenses, or of very long-term lens wear, or of very early lens wear. What I can definitely report, however, is that I am seeing a trend of younger and younger contact lens wearers presenting with symptoms of dry eye. Lens manufactur-ers have caught on to this reality as well; many are working hard to produce softer, moister-feeling, more comfortable lenses to mitigate the drying and discomfort many wearers now feel. But it would seem to make sense to alert contact lens wearers to consider reducing their wear time—alternating lenses with eye-glasses—and perhaps to undertake the environmental, nutri-tional, and lifestyle suggestions I've offered in this book, along with the self-care cleansing therapy of my Home Eye Spa pro-cedure.

Symptoms and Signs: Diagnosing Dry Eye

Diagnosing dry eye is certainly complicated by the fact that symptoms (what the patient feels) and signs (what the doctor detects on examination) very often do not correlate to one another at all. I have dealt with patients who have complained of numerous symptoms, yet the most careful and detailed exam-ination could find no cause. By the same token, I have treated patients who were entirely asymptomatic—diabetics, for exam-ple, unable to feel sensation on the eye surface—whose ocular surfaces were in fact totally scarred, dried, and irregular. And then there are those patients who complain they have the opposite of dry eye: they tear all the time. Such patients are confused to say the least by a diagnosis of dry eye—of an ocular surface so irritated that tears flow by subconscious reflex, as if the patient were cutting an onion.

Even the determination that inflammation is the likely root cause of dry eye has not solved the diagnostic problem. Inflammation also contributes to allergies and other conditions associated with dry eye, so the understanding that it is a cause of dry eye in no way clarifies or simplifies the diagnostic challenge. We must still confront symptoms and signs that can be attributed to numerous causes, or symptoms and signs that don't correlate. It means that diagnosing dry eye remains an exacting, demanding exercise that requires repeated examination and testing to puzzle out.

Still, there are more diagnostic tests available today than ever before—including my own Tear Normalization Test—and more are certainly on the way. With repeated examination and by using an array of these tests, a diagnosis of dry eye can eventually be puzzled out.

In my view, what is perhaps the toughest diagnostic nut to crack is what I refer to as the gray zone—in which individuals feel no definable symptoms but just a vague sense that something is not right. Their response to this feeling is amorphous and inarticulate; they simply cannot put a meaning to their concern, can't give it a name, and therefore can't even proceed to the idea of doing something about it.

I liken it in a way to a man with a receding hairline. He sees it; he supposes it's natural; he is aware that it is a condition that is changing his appearance. But he's not exactly racing off to the doctor for treatment.

The patient I spoke of in the Preface to this book, Bill, is a perfect example of someone in the gray zone. Bill spent a fortune on new prescription eyeglasses time after time before deciding that there might be some other explanation for his consistently deteriorating eyesight. He simply couldn't put a recognizable label on what was wrong, so he never went beyond his local "optical center" where he was given yet another short-lived improvement in visual acuity.

What people in the gray zone don't seem to know or believe is this very simple fact: difficult as it may be to name or define the discomfort, something can be done to treat it and alleviate the discomfort. There is an essential corollary to that fact: untreated, it will not get better; in fact, it will almost surely get worse.

That is why I make a fervent plea to any individual feeling any sort of eye discomfort: consider it a symptom and report it to a doctor. Chances are good that the something that can be done to alleviate the symptom is relatively simple yet can make a substantial difference. Most often, it will be something as routine as combing your hair or brushing your teeth. Incorporate such a treatment into your daily life now, when you first feel the discomfort, and you may very well stave off greater pain, more serious discomfort, and the need for more invasive medical procedures later on.

Treatment Developments

Developments in treatment modalities are making the greatest difference to dry eye sufferers today—and holding out the greatest promise for further improvements for the future. In this regard, the determination that inflammation is the primary cause of dry eye has been critical, and it has spawned an entire new family of pharmaceutical treatments.

But perhaps as important is the understanding about the impact of environmental factors, nutrition, and lifestyle behaviors. Among my patients, I find that the program outlined in Part Two of this book makes a profound difference in the way they look, feel, and see. Certainly, all of the recommendations in the program apply for overall health as well: omega-3 fatty acids, untroubled sleep, exercise, stress reduction, and the like benefit the general population as well as the population of dry eye sufferers. But the difference it can make to the comfort level of the latter can be dramatic; I've seen it with my own eyes.

One caveat: patience and perseverance may be needed before that dramatic difference is felt and recognized. I've had patients who swore to me they were following the recommendations but reported no change in their symptoms for four, five, even six visits to my office. Then suddenly they'll announce: "You know, I'm feeling much better." So it is well worth persisting in these environmental, nutritional, and lifestyle adjustments; sooner or later, the difference will be felt.

But certainly, the most exciting news on the treatment front today is coming from the pharmaceutical companies, and they deserve the gratitude of all dry eye sufferers for responding to the needs of the marketplace and giving this disorder the attention it merits. At least a dozen new drugs are currently in development and testing, ready for release to the market some time around 2010 to 2015. What is particularly exciting about these products is that they represent a range of approaches. Some are hormonal, inspired by findings that an androgen deficiency may lead to dry eye. Some are anti-inflammatory medications used for other conditions and now being converted to ophthalmic use. Some attempt to re-create the natural human tear film. The bottom line is a growing array of more and more options for those who suffer from dry eye.

Hope For the Future: Therapies 'In the Pipeline'

Here's a look at some of those options. Below are therapies now in the pipeline—that is, in various phases of testing as they make their way, hopefully, to the marketplace.

Keep in mind that clinical testing can last for years. Typically, phase I looks at safety issues, phase II at effectiveness, and phase III at benefits, risks, and possible side effects. But these phases can often overlap. The real distinction between phases is the number of people involved in the trials: each succeeding phase will involve increasingly greater numbers; phase III testing typically involves many thousands of people with the condition the therapy is intended to benefit. And of course, there is laboratory testing that happens even before a therapy is ready for clinical testing.

Bottom line? The process can take time, but it does eventually produce new therapies that have been comprehensively tested and found to work. Here are the most promising therapies in the pipeline for dry eye sufferers (in order by how close they are to FDA approval):

Diquafasol (Inspire Pharmaceuticals): Stimulates goblet cell mucus secretion and the watery component, thus improving multiple components of the tear film-awaiting FDA approval.

SPHP 700 (Sinclair Pharma): Uses natural polysaccharide combined with a polymer to provide prolonged wetting—approved for use in Europe, expected on the U.S. market as prescription drop in 2007.

Rebamipide (Otsuka): Increases mucus secretion—in phase III clinical testing, may be one of the first to surface in near future.

Nova 22007 (Novagali): A cyclosporine anti-inflammatory emulsion, somewhat similar to Restasis—recently started phase III testing.

Pimecrolimus (Novartis): Anti-inflammatory eye drop that will address the source of dry eye—completed phase II testing, soon beginning phase III.

Ecabet (ISTA): Increases mucus secretion; may be the first drop to address both the signs and symptoms of dry eye—completed phase II testing, will start phase III testing in 2007.

NP 50301 (Nascent): Estrogen topical eye drop developed by Aborn with funding from Nascent to address hormone deficiencies—completed phase II testing, soon to start Phase III testing.

Testosterone eye cream (Southern College of Optometry and Argentis)—in advanced clinical testing, could be on the market soon.

Androgen Tears (Allergan): Testosterone drops—finished phase II testing, has a very promising future but may be many years away.

Moli 1901 (Lantibio): Used typically for cystic fibrosis by hydrating the lining of the lung epithelium, facilitating the removal of mucus secretions, and could hydrate the ocular surface in dry eye patients—in Phase II testing.

Rimexolone (Alcon): Steroid eye drop used for other conditions that may prove useful in decreasing the inflammation associated with dry eyes—in Phase II testing.

CF-101 (Can-Fite Biopharma): Anti-inflammatory agent—completed Phase II-A trials for treating rheumatoid arthritis and soon to be tested for dry eyes.

15-(S)-HETE (Alcon): Eye drop that increases mucus secretion—has had difficulty in proving efficacy in its late-phase testing.

Alacrity ALTY-0501 (BioScience): Topical doxycycline product that entered phase II trials in late 2006.

Estratest (Solvay): Oral estrogen and testosterone used as hormone replacement therapy for other conditions—about to start clinical trials for dry eye treatment.

Cevilamine (Daiichi): Stimulates water layer secretion—in Phase II trials.

Milcrin (VISTA): Has mucus-like characteristics, would be used to simulate mucus—in early stages of development.

Trehalose (Biovision): Found in the skin of desert reptiles, which it seems to keep moist; thus may help human eyes to retain moisture—awaiting testing.

D-B-Hydroxybutyrate (Ophtecs Corporation): May protect the ocular surface by protecting against early skin cell death—in early testing.

Lacritin (Senju): Topical treatment based in the protein, lacritin, that has been found to be deficient in patients with blepharitis; promotes tear production—in early testing.

Because so many dry eye sufferers are post-menopausal women, the hormone-based therapies may offer hope for the most dramatic improvement in the condition—simply by dint of the numbers of people that would be affected. As research continues to address the relationship between hormones and the ocular surface, it's increasingly likely science will discover the exact nature of that relationship—whether androgen-based, estrogen-based, or a combination of those factors. That's why this research is so promising.

Offering even further hope to dry eye sufferers is the reality that the more products there are, the more the competition intensifies; this spawns yet more products—and conceivably brings down their price. That alone can aid compliance by patients, but equally important in that regard are efforts to ease the regimens under which medications must be taken. If, for example, I as a doctor could prescribe an affordable medication a patient would need to take only once a day to alleviate the symptoms of dry eye, I would have a lot more confidence that the patient would stick to that regimen and improve the long-term health of his or her eyes. And who can say what the impact of that might be on the individual's productivity in the work-place and safety behind the wheel?

For the moment, however, there are plenty of treatment options to choose from. As dry eye sufferers look to the prom-ise of many more options to come—even, perhaps, to a total therapeutic cure—there is no reason they shouldn't do so through refreshed, clear, comfortably moist eyes.

RESOURCES

MORE INFORMATION ON DRY EYE

The Dry Eye Center of New York

115 East 57th Street, 10th floor

New York, NY 10022

212-832-2020

220 Westchester Avenue West

White Plains, NY 10604-2913

914-328-5300

www.dryeyedoctor.com

Dr. Robert Latkany's medical offices and website offer information about the causes and treatments of dry eye, as well as products that can help relieve dry eye and opportunities to participate in clinical trials of new dry eye treatments.

AgingEye Times

PMB # 234

1 Kendall Square

Cambridge, MA 02139

www.agingeye.net

This comprehensive website, affiliated with University of Illinois at Chicago, addresses diseases of the aging eye, including a good section on dry eyes.

The Dry Eye Company

PO Box 3447

Apollo Beach, FL 33572

877-693-7939

www.dryeyezone.com

This website gathers the latest information and offers an online chat room where dry eye sufferers can share experiences.

EMedicine

Omaha, NE

402-341-3222

www.emedicinehealth.com

This general health website, affiliated with WebMD, includes a good section on dry eye syndrome.

Focus on Dry Eye

www.chronicdryeye.com

This site, sponsored by Allergan, includes articles and videos explaining symptoms and treatments for dry eye.

National Eye Institute

Building 31, Room 6A32

31 Center Drive, MSC 2510

Bethesda, MD 20892

301-496-5248

www.nei.nih.gov/health/cornealdisease/index.asp

www.nei.nih.gov/health/blepharitis/index.asp

These two government sites are excellent sources for a thorough understanding of dry eye.

National Women's Health Resource Center

157 Broad Street, Suite 315

Red Bank, NJ 07701

877-986-9472

www.healthywomen.org

In addition to a comprehensive dry eye section under Health Topics, you can search this site for tips, articles, Q&A, fact-sheets, late-breaking news.

Office on Women's Health

U.S. Department of Health and Human Services

800-994-9662

www.womenshealth.gov

Federal government source for information on women's health. Search for "dry eye" to come up with current thinking, reports on the latest research, and suggestions for treatment.

Sjögren's Syndrome Foundation

8120 Woodmont Avenue, Suite 530

Bethesda, MD 20814-1437

800-475-6473

www.Sjögrens.org

Foundation and website devoted to this very common cause of severe dry eye.

Society for Women's Health Research

1025 Connecticut Avenue, NW, Suite 701

Washington, DC 20036

202-223-8224

www.womenshealthresearch.org

The nation's only nonprofit dedicated to improving the health of all women through research, education, and advocacy. Has paid particularly close attention to dry eyes and is a good search engine on the topic.

St. Luke's Tarpon Springs

43309 U.S. Hwy 19N

Tarpon Springs, FL 34689

800-282-9905

www.stlukeseye.com

Check this website for excellent information on eye disorders in general and dry eye syndrome in particular.

RELATED MEDICAL CONDITIONS

DIABETES

An estimated half of diabetics suffer from dry eye.

American Diabetes Association

1701 North Beauregard Street

Alexandria, VA 22311

800-342-2383

www.diabetes.org

RHEUMATOID ARTHRITIS

Rheumatoid arthritis is one form of arthritis; those who suffer from it will also experience dry eye.

American College of Rheumatology Research and Education Foundation

1800 Century Place, Suite 250

Atlanta, GA 30345-4300

404-633-3777

www.rheumatology.org

ROSACEA

Most patients with rosacea have ocular rosacea, with associated blephar-itis, meibomian gland dysfunction, and dry eye. The following associa-tions offer information and help.

International Rosacea Foundation

www.internationalrosaceafoundation.org

National Rosacea Society

800 S. Northwest Hwy., Suite 200

Barrington, IL 60010

888-NOBLUSH (888 662-5874)

www.rosacea.org

The Rosacea Research & Development Institute

PO Box 234

Pandora, OH 45877

www.irosacea.org

Rosacea Support Group

www.rosacea.ii.net

SJÖGREN'S SYNDROME

As many as four million Americans suffer from this condition that typically presents with dry skin, dry eye, arthritis, and dry mouth. This is the
signature website for the disease.

Sjögren's Syndrome Foundation

8120 Woodmont Avenue, Suite 530

Bethesda, MD 20814-1437

800-475-6473

www.Sjögrens.org

STEVENS JOHNSON SYNDROME

Stevens Johnson is a debilitating condition that typically leaves patients
with chronic scarring and severe dry eye.

Stevens Johnson Syndrome Foundation

PO Box 350333

Westminster, CO 80035-0333

303-635-1241

www.sjsupport.org

THYROID DISORDER

Any thyroid disorder can cause or exacerbate dry eye.

The Thyroid Foundation of America
One Longfellow Place, Suite 1518

Boston, MA 02114

800 832-8321

www.tsh.org

EYE DROPS

ADVANCED EYE RELIEF, LOTEMAX, AND ALREX
Bausch & Lomb

1 Bausch & Lomb Place

Rochester, NY 14604

585-338-6000

www.bausch.com/en_US/consumer/consumer_home.aspx

Bausch & Lomb offers over-the-counter Advanced Eye Relief artificial tear products and the low-potency topical steroid drops, Lotemax and Alrex.

GENTEAL AND HYPOTEARS

Novartis Pharmaceuticals Corporation

Customer Interaction Center

One Health Plaza

East Hanover, NJ 07936–1080

1-888-NOW-NOVA (1-888-669-6682)

www.us.novartisophthalmics.com/index.jsp

Novartis manufactures two brands of over-the-counter artificial tears, Gen-Teal and HypoTears. Most of the GenTeal products contain a disappearing preservative to minimize irritation; GenTeal PF is preservative-free.

MINIDROPS EYE THERAPY

Optics Laboratory Inc.

9480 Telstar Avenue, Suite 3

El Monte, CA 91731

800-968-6788

www.minidrops.com

MiniDrops are preservative-free artificial tears.

NATURE'S TEARS EYEMIST

Nature's Tears

Bio-Logics Aqua Technologies

PO Box 400

Grants Pass, OR 97528

800-367-6478

www.naturestears.com

Nature's Tears is a non-allergenic, preservative-free spray moisturizer for the eyes for those patients who are averse to using eye drops.

RESTASIS AND REFRESH

Allergan, Inc.

PO Box 19534

Irvine, CA 92623

714-246-4500

www.allergan.com

Allergan is the maker of prescription-only Restasis and all over-the-counter Refresh artificial tear products.

SOOTHE EMOLLIENT (LUBRICANT) EYE DROPS

Alimera Sciences

6120 Windward Parkway, Suite 290

Alpharetta, GA 30005

678-990-5740

www.alimerasciences.com

Soothe is the first multi-dose lubricant eye drop to feature Restoryl, a unique lipid restorative that works to re-establish the lipid (oily) layer of tears to last up to 8 hours!

SYSTANE, TEARS NATURALE, AND BION

Alcon

6201 South Freeway

Fort Worth, TX 76134-2099

www.alconlabs.com

Alcon currently produces Systane, Tears Naturale, and Bion over-the-counter artificial tear products but is focusing primarily on its newest line, Systane Lubricant Eye Drops, which is longer lasting.

THERATEARS

Advanced Vision Research

660 Main Street

Woburn, MA 01801

800-979-8327

www.theratears.com

TheraTears products contain a patented electrolyte composition that precisely matches the human tear film.

OMEGA-3 FATTY ACID SUPPLEMENTS

DRY-VITES

Deep Blue See

PO Box 373

Rye, NY 10580

212-832-2020

www.deepbluesee.net

My own company, Deep Blue See, distributes Dry-Vites, which consist solely of wild salmon oil and flaxseed oil. Because the salmon is wild and short-lived, its oil is less likely to have impurities. And because there are no vitamins present in the product, Dry-Vites can be taken with other supplements and medications.

HYDROEYE

ScienceBased Health

3579 Highway 50 East

Carson City, NV 89701

888-433-4726

www.sciencebasedhealth.com

HydroEye is a combination of many ingredients, including omega-3s from black currant seed oil and a small amount of cod liver oil; it also has a high vitamin A content. Another established product.

THERATEARS NUTRITION

Advanced Vision Research

660 Main Street

Woburn, MA 01801

800-979-8327

www.theratears.com

TheraTears Nutrition, composed of marine lipid oil, flaxseed oil, and vitamin E, is a product that has been on the market for some time and is well established.

ZOOMEGA-3

Biosyntrx

151A Riverchase Way

Lexington, SC 29072

800-688-6815

www.biosyntrx.com

ZoOmega-3, another well established product, comes from Biosyntrx. It gets its omega-3s from a high concentration of cod liver oil and a smaller concentration of black currant seed oil—and contains other ingredients as well.

EYE CARE PRODUCTS

DEEP BLUE SEE

PO Box 373

Rye, NY 10580

212-832-2020

www.deepbluesee.net

Supplements, heating eye pads, cooling eye pads, pocket-sized insulated carrying bags to keep eye drops cool, tranquileyes goggles for nighttime lagophthalmos relief are all provided through my own company, Deep Blue See.

VISIONS EYE CENTER

117 Decatur Street, Suite 1

Brooklyn, NY 11216

www.comfortableeyes.com

A variety of eye products, such as drops and goggles, is available via this website.

BOSTON FOUNDATION FOR SIGHT

464 Hillside Avenue, Suite 205

Needham, MA 02494

781-726-7333

www.bostonsight.org

The Boston scleral lens, a prosthetic device like a contact lens that rests on the white of the eye and holds a reservoir of artificial tears over the cornea, can be obtained here. The Boston Foundation for Sight is a 501(c)2 nonprofit and provides free and subsidized care to qualified patients. Further information is available on the website.

EYEECO

Murietta, CA

888-730-7999

www.eyeeco.com

Eyeeco created and distributes tranquileyes, the nighttime goggles.

LEITER'S PHARMACY

1700 Park Avenue, Suite 30

San Jose, CA 95126

800-292-6773

408-292-6772

408-288-8252 (fax)

http://www.leiterrx.com/index.html

Virtually any eye drop you take can be made into a preservative-free product that will be shipped the next day—guaranteed—by this specialized pharmacy.

OCUSOFT

PO Box 429

Richmond, TX 77406

800 233-5469

http://www.ocusoft.com

Eyelid scrubs for blepharitis sufferers can be found at this site.

PANOPTX

1252 Quarry Lane

Pleasanton, CA 94566

925-484-0292

http://www.panoptx.com

Panoptx eyewear provides moisture chamber goggles and filtered vents.

PUNCTAL PLUGS

The following companies supply various types, sizes, and shapes of punctal plugs. A doctor can insert the plugs via a minor procedure done in the doctor's office and typically covered by your insurance. Punctal plugs help dry eye sufferers keep their own tears in their eyes longer.

EAGLE VISION, INC.

8500 Wolf Lake Drive, Suite 110

PO Box 34877

Memphis, TN 38184

800-222-7584

www.dryeye.org

FCI-OPHTHALMICS

P.O. Box 465

Marshfield Hills, MA 02051

800-932-4202

www.fci-ophthalmics.com

MEDENNIUM, INC.

9 Parker, Suite 150

Irvine, CA 92618

888-727-6100

www.medennium.com

OASIS MEDICAL INC.

510-528 South Vermont Avenue

Glendora, CA 91741

800-528-9786

www.oasismedical.com

ODYSSEY

5828 Shelby Oaks Dr.

Memphis, TN 38134

888-905-7770

www.odysseymed.com

INDEX

VISION TEST

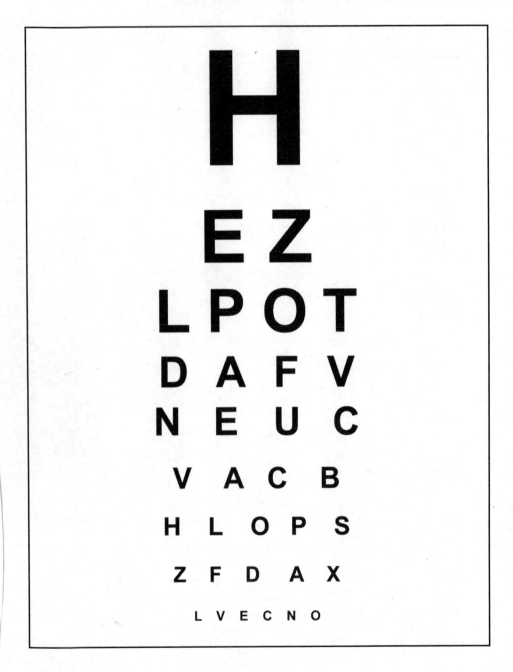